IDENTITY, GENDER, AND SEXUALITY

CONTROVERSIES IN PSYCHOANALYSIS SERIES

IDENTITY, GENDER, AND SEXUALITY
150 Years after Freud

Edited by

Peter Fonagy, Rainer Krause,
Marianne Leuzinger-Bohleber

Foreword by

Cláudio Laks Eizirik

Controversies in Psychoanalysis Series

Routledge
Taylor & Francis Group
LONDON AND NEW YORK

Figure 3.1 (p. 67) reprinted from *Bright Air, Brilliant Fire* by Gerald Edelman (New York: Basic Books, 1992; Harmondsworth: Penguin, 1994), p. 84, by permission of The Perseus Books Group, New York, and Penguin UK.

"Colin's Story" (pp. 125–129) reprinted with permission from "The etiology of boyhood gender identity disorder: A model for integrating psychodynamics, temperament and development", by S. Coates, R. Friedman, & S. Wolfe; *Psychoanalytic Dialogues, 1* (1991): 481–523; The Analytic Press Publishers.

First published in 2006 by
The International Psychoanalytical Association

First published 2009 by Karnac Books Ltd.

Published 2019 by Routledge
2 Park Square, Milton Park, Abingdon, Oxon OX14 4RN
52 Vanderbilt Avenue, New York, NY 10017

First issued in hardback 2019

Routledge is an imprint of the Taylor & Francis Group, an informa business

British Library Cataloguing in Publication Data
A C.I.P. for this book is available from the British Library

ISBN 13: 978-0-367-10671-3 (hbk)
ISBN 13: 978-1-85575-764-6 (pbk)

Edited, designed, and produced by Communication Crafts

CONTENTS

CONTROVERSIES IN PSYCHOANALYSIS SERIES

IPA Publications Committee

The present Publications Committee of the International Psychoanalytical Association initiates, with this volume, a new series, *Controversies in Psychoanalysis*, the objective of which is to reflect, within the frame of our publishing policy, present debates and polemics in the psychoanalytic field.

Theoretical and clinical progress in psychoanalysis continues to develop new concepts and to reconsider old ones, often in contradiction with each other.

By confronting and opening these debates, we might find points of convergence but also divergences that cannot be reconciled; the ensuing tension among these should be sustained in a pluralistic dialogue.

This series will focus on these complex intersections through various thematic proposals developed by authors from within different theoretical frameworks and from diverse geographical areas, in order to open possibilities of generating a productive debate within the psychoanalytic world and related professional circles.

We are pleased to begin this series with the support of Cláudio Eizirik, President of the International Psychoanalytical Association. Special thanks are due to the editors, Peter Fonagy, Rainer Krause, and Marianne Leuzinger-Bohleber, and to the contributors to this first volume. We are also grateful to the former Publications Committee and their chair, Emma Piccioli, under whose mandate this volume was first commissioned.

Leticia Glocer Fiorini
Chair of the Publications Committee

ACKNOWLEDGEMENTS

We would like to express our thanks and gratitude to many colleagues who have given us support and helpful critique in writing and publishing this book: particularly to Cesare Sacerdoti and Emma Piccioli from the former Publications Committee of the International Psychoanalytical Association, and Klara and Eric King of Communication Crafts. Without their professionalism, engagement, and careful work—in spite of all the time pressure—this book would not have been published. We also thank Marion Ebert-Saleh and Herbert Bareuther, from the Sigmund-Freud-Institute, Frankfurt, who carefully edited first versions of the manuscripts and organized the bibliographies.

The contributions to this book are modified papers that were given at the Sixth Joseph Sandler Research Conference in March 2005 at University College London, which was devoted to the 100th anniversary of Freud's *Three Essays on the Theory of Sexuality* (1905d). The papers had been of such high quality that we decided to publish them in this book. We hope that this volume may inspire us to estimate anew Freud's most innovative discoveries on this topic, as well as to develop further the insights collected in this clinically still most relevant field, integrating results from psychoanalytic and non-psychoanalytic studies during the last century of exciting research.

Peter Fonagy, Rainer Krause, Marianne Leuzinger-Bohleber

ABOUT THE EDITORS AND CONTRIBUTORS

Susan Coates (New York) is an Associate Clinical Professor of Psychology in the Department of Psychiatry, College of Physicians and Surgeons, Columbia University, where she is on the faculty of The Columbia Center for Psychoanalytic Training and Research and also teaches in its Parent–Infant Program. She is the editor, with Jane Rosenthal and Dan Schechter, of the book *September 11: Trauma and Human Bonds*. She is on several editorial boards, including *The Journal of Infant, Child and Adolescent Psychotherapy*; *Studies in Gender and Sexuality*: and the Italian journal *Infanzia e Adolescenza*. She has published extensively on issues of gender, trauma, and attachment in young children.

Peter Fonagy (London) is Freud Memorial Professor of Psychoanalysis and Director of the Sub-Department of Clinical Health Psychology at University College London. He is Chief Executive of the Anna Freud Centre, London, and Consultant to the Child and Family Program at the Menninger Department of Psychiatry at Baylor College of Medicine. He is a clinical psychologist and a training and super ising analyst in the British Psychoanalytical Society in child and adult analysis. He holds a number of important positions, which include

Co-Chairing the Research Committee of the International Psychoanalytical Association and Fellowship of the British Academy.

Richard C. Friedman (New York) is Clinical Professor of Psychiatry at Well Medical College (Cornell), Lecturer in Psychiatry at Columbia, and Professor at The Derner Institute, Adelphi University. He is the author of *Male Homosexuality: A Contemporary Psychoanalytic Perspective* (1988). Recently he has published many articles on sexual orientation with Jennifer Downey; their article on female homosexuality received an award from *The Journal of the American Psychoanalytic Association* as the journal's best publication of 1997. Friedman and Downey's most recent book is *Sexual Orientation and Psychoanalysis: Sexual Science and Clinical Practice* (published in 2002).

André E. Haynal (Geneva) is Honorary Professor and former Chairman of the Department of Psychiatry, University of Geneva, and former Visiting Professor at Stanford University in California. He is also a former President of the Swiss Psychoanalytic Society and a former Vice-President of the European Psychoanalytical Federation. He is author of nine books (the originals in French) and many publications—among others, *Depression and Creativity*; *Fanaticism*; *The Technique at Issue: Controversies in Psychoanalysis, from Freud and Ferenczi to Michael Balint*; *Disappearing and Reviving: Sándor Ferenczi in the History of Psychoanalysis*—and scientific editor of the *Freud/Ferenczi Correspondence.*

Rainer Krause is Professor of Clinical Psychology and Psychotherapy and Dean of the Faculty of Empirical Life Sciences, University of the Saarland. He is a member of the Swiss Psychoanalytic Society and the German Psychoanalytical Society, DPG. He is also a training analyst and founder of the Saarland Psychoanalytic Institute, and his research is on affect and affect exchange processes as they form transference and countertransference processes.

Marianne Leuzinger-Bohleber is a training analyst in the German Psychoanalytical Association, a member of the Swiss Psychoanalytical Society, professor for psychoanalytic psychology at the University of Kassel, and Head Director of the Sigmund-Freud-Institute, Frankfurt. Her main research fields include epistemology and methods of clinical and empirical research in psychoanalysis; interdisciplinary discourse with embodied cognitive science, and modern German literature.

Linda C. Mayes (New Haven/London) is the Arnold Gesell Professor of Child Psychiatry, Pediatrics, and Psychology in the Yale Child Study Center. She is also chairman of the directorial team of the Anna Freud Centre and a member of the faculty of the Western New England Psychoanalytic Institute in New Haven, Connecticut. She has been a member of the faculty of Yale University School of Medicine since 1985. She trained as both a child and adult psychoanalyst and as a paediatrician, neonatologist, and child developmentalist; her work integrates perspectives from developmental psychology, neuroscience, and child psychiatry. Her scientific papers and chapters are published in the child psychiatric, developmental psychology, paediatric, and psychoanalytic literature.

Friedemann Pfäfflin (Ulm) is Professor of Psychotherapy, University Clinic of Psychosomatic Medicine and Psychotherapy, Forensic Psychotherapy Section, University of Ulm, Germany. From 1978 to1992 he worked in the Department of Sex Research, Psychiatric University Clinic, Hamburg. He is a psychiatrist and training analyst of the German Psychoanalytical Association. He is past President of the Harry Benjamin International Gender Dysphoria Association, Inc. (HBIGDA), past President of the International Association for Forensic Psychotherapy (IAFP), and is President of the International Association for the Treatment of Sexual Offenders (IATSO).

Anne-Marie Sandler (London) was born in Geneva, studied with Jean Piaget, and was, for a time, his assistant. She then came to England, where she trained in child analysis with Anna Freud, going on to complete the adult training in the British Psychoanalytical Society, where she is a training and supervising analyst. She has been President of the British Society and of the European Psychoanalytical Federation and Vice-President of the International Psychoanalytical Association. She was formerly Director of the Anna Freud Centre. Many of her published papers were written in collaboration with Joseph Sandler. They also collaborated on a book, *Internal Objects Revisited* (published in 1998).

Sheila Spensley (London) is now retired but was formerly a consultant clinical psychologist in London. She has had many years' experience of working psychoanalytically with psychotic adults and children. She also trained in both child and adult psychotherapy at the Tavistock Clinic. Currently she is involved in the training of child psychotherapists and is researching mother–child attachment relationships where the child has a major learning difficulty. Her publications have focused on the interface of psychotic and autistic pathology and its developmental implications.

Sverre Varvin (Oslo) works in private practice and is senior researcher at the Norwegian Centre for Violence and Traumatic Stress Studies. He is a member and training analyst of the Norwegian Psychoanalytic Society, a member of the committee on conceptual research in the International Psychoanalytical Association, and chair of the working group on trauma of the European Psychoanalytical Federation. His research interests include traumatization, psychotherapy with traumatized patients, process-outcome research in psychoanalysis, and qualitative research.

Rudi Vermote (Brussels) is a psychoanalyst of the Belgian Society for Psychoanalysis in private practice. As a psychiatrist he is head of the Hospitalization-Based Psychotherapy Unit at the University Centre, Kortenberg, Belgium, and lecturer in the psychotherapy training at the University of Leuven. He is an IPA Research Fellow and conducted a process-outcome study on the treatment of personality disorders. He is editor of the *Revue Belge de Psychanalyse* and of the *Tijdschrift voor Psychoanalyse* and *Psychoanalytisch Actueel*. He has an interest in applied psychoanalysis and has written papers on the application of Bion's ideas in the field of personality disorders, psychosis, mental retardation, and multiple sclerosis.

FOREWORD

Cláudio Laks Eizirik

I am very pleased to welcome the new IPA's Publications Committee Series *Controversies in Psychoanalysis* and to congratulate the Committee and its chair, Leticia Glocer Fiorini.

In the year in which we celebrate Freud's 150th birthday, several meetings have been organized in different regions and societies, not only to celebrate, but mainly to evaluate, discuss, and propose new directions to the seminal insights of the creator of psychoanalysis. There is little room nowadays for dogmatic, simply exegetic, and repetitive approaches in any field of knowledge. What we need are new perspectives, lively views, and open debate on so many controversial areas of science and the humanities. Being part of both realms of knowledge, psychoanalysis naturally welcomes an approach to the main controversies in its theory, practice, and application to other fields.

Identity, Gender and Sexuality: 150 Years after Freud, edited by Peter Fonagy, Rainer Krause, and Marianne Leuzinger-Bohleber, is an important contribution to one of the most controversial themes since the very beginning of psychoanalysis. A century ago, when Freud's *Three Essays on the Theory of Sexuality* (1905d) was published, the reception was initially negative, but it did not take many years for the acknowledgement that that book offered a revolutionary set of insights that changed forever the way we understand and approach the many dimensions of human sexuality. From then on, however, several new concepts and ways of understanding normal and pathological expressions of sexuality appeared, as well as new data from child observation, clinical experiences, and empirical and conceptual research. In this "sexual century", as Ethel Person has called it, psychoanalysis has learned much and witnessed new contributions that enable us not only to understand better, but also to treat with greater accuracy, various kinds of sexual expressions, behaviours, and feelings.

This book is a very good beginning for the new series, and I am sure that subsequent titles will continue to offer such a stimulating source of information, updated concepts, and the sort of intellectual challenges that make us always so eager to be part of this fascinating work in progress that can only grow through real controversies.

1

Psychosexuality and psychoanalysis: an overview

Peter Fonagy

The 1997 Congress of the International Psychoanalytic in Barcelona was spent discussing the relationship of psychoanalysis with sexuality. The title of the Congress—"Psychoanalysis *and* Sexuality"—already indicated that psychoanalysis and sexuality *could* be considered separately (Stein, 1998b). I doubt that the title would have made sense to the psychoanalysts of the pioneering, heroic generation. But the title reflected something real about the current status of sexuality in our theory and practice. It is as if there is no space for sexuality within psychoanalysis. We no longer consider it fundamental in all cases or even relevant to current theorization. I am reminded of a famous Victorian, who commented dismissively about sex: "The position is ludicrous, the pleasure is momentary, and the expense damnable." Freud's discoveries are an emblem, a symbol of a worthy tradition, but of little actual relevance to clinical understanding or practice. Ruth Stein (1998b) put it thus: "Freud's early insight that diverse psychic phenomena, contents and symptoms are expressions of defences against sexual, mostly oedipal, themes has taken its full swing on the dialectical pendulum of psychoanalytic thinking" (p. 254). Psychosexuality is nowadays more frequently considered as disguising other, non-sexual self- and object-related conflicts than the other way round.

Why has sex moved out of psychoanalysis?

Some still insist that the hallmark of psychoanalysis is its concern with sexuality (Green, 1995, 1997b; Spruiell, 1997). Yet it is an open secret that this cannot be the case. Current major theories of psychoanalysis, including object-relations theory, self psychology, and intersubjective relational approaches, perhaps with the exception of the French school, place the crux of their clinical accounts elsewhere—principally in the relationship domain. We have undertaken a survey of the use of sexual and relational language in the electronically searchable journals of psychoanalysis. In brief, we have noted a dramatic decline in words in psychoanalytic articles that directly concern sexuality (words for sexual body parts, sexual orientation, normative and non-normative sexual behaviours), as well as theoretical language concerning the sexual, referring to metapsychology or oral, anal, or genital sexuality. Interestingly, contrasting this decline with relational theoretical words—such as attachment, attunement, object seeking, object relations—indicates that the decline is not of jargon words but specific to sexual theoretical language. Even contrasting general relational words—such as love, affection, intimacy, kindness, affiliation, relatedness, connectedness—with general sexual words referring to body parts, orientation, and sexual acts shows the asymmetry between the two domains. Thus, although we may pay lip service to the continued importance of sexuality and use vociferous rhetoric to assert its primacy in our thinking, our writings and probably our daily practice belie this.

There is no shortage of explanation as to why this might have occurred. It might help to contextualize our arguments if we consider a few. Perhaps the most significant issue concerns the intimate link between *drive theory* and *psychosexuality*. Traditionally, sexuality has been held to illustrate and in most respects to be essentially equated with the drives (e.g. Rapaport, 1960). In some ways, it might appear that psychosexuality exits with classical metapsychology. The link, however, remains firm in many minds. For example, Green suggests that: "*human sexuality is characterised mainly by the constancy of the pressure of the sex drive which is not limited to periods of 'heat' as in animals*" (Green, 1997b, pp. 349–350; italics in original). Yet, in drive-theory accounts, the intensity of sexuality is seen reductively as being due to the force of drives. Paradoxically, in classical theory, sexuality is nothing special: its psychic potency is fully accounted for by its direct connection with the drives. In mixed drive-theory and object-relations accounts such as Kernberg's (1976, 1992), the model becomes somewhat more complex but essentially remains the same: the intensity associated with sexuality is attributed to primitive object relations that are, in their turn, imbued with developmentally less well integrated and therefore more intense affect states. In addition to being reductive, the equation of the developmentally early, with more experientially intense and disturbing, may be a convenient metaphor but rests on shaky conceptual and empirical foundations (Westen, 1997; Willick, 2001).

There is also the classical account proposing *resistance*. Psychoanalysts may not be immune to the forces of repression that push infantile sexuality out of consciousness in all our lives. Can the reduction of psychoanalytic interest in the sexual be a consequence of common-or-garden resistance? Freud anticipated resistance to psychosexuality, particularly its infantile aspects, and this, more than any other aspect of the theory, has been viewed as explaining the unpalatability of psychoanalysis in general (Spruiell, 1997). The expected objection to this account entails the shift in the public perception of sexuality. It was easier to mount this argument 100 years ago, when main-line culture was dystonic with human sexuality. Currently, sexuality is more than ever at the forefront of individual consciousness and is an important vehicle for the support of the social institutions we charge with the dissemination of our ideas: the media.

Perhaps paradoxically, there is more evidence of psychoanalysts seeming eager, at least unconsciously, to erase psychosexuality than Western culture as a whole. There is, and there has always been, considerable *prudishness about sexual practices* in psychoanalytic public debate and in (certainly British) clinical discussions of individual cases. In the immediate post-Freudian years there was an absence of cultural relativity in discussions of sex and an authoritarian imposition of oedipal genital sexuality as a gold standard for psychological health. A very dramatic illustration of the denial of sexuality by psychoanalysts was the resistance to recognizing the prevalence of sexual abuse of children by the very profession that put childhood sexuality on the scientific map of the psyche. These forces may have served to "inhibit" the psychoanalytic study of sexuality.

The importance that twentieth-century culture attaches to sexuality may have played a part in the reduced attention psychoanalysts nowadays pay to the sexual aspects of mental life. Analysts felt tarred with the brush of *pansexualism.* The reservations about making psychosexuality the background and basis of psychoanalysis grew, perhaps alongside (or as a result of) patients' conscious expectation of sexual interpretations by analysts. The very popularity of the psychoanalytic movement inoculated analytic patients against simplistic sexual interpretations. The profound gender bias of Freudian psychosexual theory also jarred in the context of the feminist enlightenment of the second half of the twentieth century.

Another consideration to which André Green (1997a, 1997b) draws attention is the rise of *developmental theory,* particularly the introduction and general acceptance of fundamentally Kleinian ideas. Melanie Klein reinterpreted phallic and genital sexuality in terms of an earlier libidinal stage and understood the psychosexual as primarily recreating patterns of infantile relationships to the breast. Even though Klein and her followers conceived of this as a simple extension of Freud's ideas, the relation between the part-object of the drive (the breast) and its corresponding erotogenic zone (the mouth) came to be linked with the relationship of the infant to the whole object (the mother). This perspective, historically, led to a focus on the relationship between self and object that could not be reduced to a notion of an object as non-particular and interchangeable with any other object that could fulfil the same function for that drive. Developmentalists are frequently blamed for diverting psychoanalytic attention from sexuality. In my view this is the opposite of the truth: *observations of infant development will provide the long-awaited model of human sexuality that psychoanalysis has missed since its inception.*

Perhaps a less complex account may be given in terms of the shifting clinical interests of psychoanalysts. With the emergence of cheaper and shorter interventions, both pharmacological and psychotherapeutic, for the simple, relatively quickly reversible, episodic—"neurotic"—disorders, psychoanalysis inevitably became a treatment option for more enduring personality problems such as narcissism, borderline personality disorder, and the more characterological end of the mood disorders. Not that sexuality plays no part in the life of such individuals. But, as Herbert Rosenfeld (1952) was perhaps the first to point out, for many of these patients interpretations involving sexuality were not only unhelpful but were often taken almost as suggestions of sexual activity by the analysts and caused considerable complications. I vividly remember my first analytic experience with a borderline patient. Early in his analysis, following a lengthy discussion of his anxieties concerning competitiveness, I ventured to point out that these might be related to unresolved conflicts about his sexual competition with his father as a little boy (I am still ashamed of the degree of my naiveté). He seemed thoughtful about my interpretation and returned proudly the following day with an account of a dream where he and his father were fighting; he had a knife, and after a struggle managed to cut his father's penis off, which he held up victoriously, reminding himself of the Statue of Liberty. By then I had the presence of mind to make the more appropriate interpretation that his anxiety the day before concerned his feeling of being in competition with me, and now, having witnessed my inadequacy, he could, indeed, afford to feel triumphant.

Implicit in these clinical observations is the idea that in disorders where ego functioning is at the centre of the pathology, even pathological sexuality has to be understood in terms of some other structure that subsumes it. The paradigm shift in psychoanalysis, which led to the emphasis on object relations, may at first sight appear to have precluded serious consideration of psychosexuality. Object-relations explanations have, at least in part, been inspired by observations of mother–infant interactions, which have been suggested to preclude serious consideration being given to "the intrapsychic consequences of the sexual drives that do not readily lend themselves to observation" (Green, 1997b, p. 347). In particular, attachment theory, which has—at least in recent years—been extremely influential in the evolution of psychoanalytic object-relations ideas, avoids consideration of the psychosexual aspects of attachment. This seems to be more a question of preference than of necessity, as many object-relations models have contributed to the understanding of sexuality (e.g. Kernberg, 1992). Perhaps it is the historical association of psychosexuality with drive theory, which remains an anathema to many object-relations theorists, that accounts for the decoupling of sexuality and attachment. This is all the more puzzling since normal sexual behaviour quite evidently incorporates aspects of the mother–infant relationship. Yet within an object-relations framework, most often sexual material, whether in the transference, in free association, or in dreams, is interpreted as defensive against a presumed underlying relationship-based pathology: for example, excitement created to ward off annihilation anxiety, or sex to perform manic reparation and deny guilt over destructiveness. Sexual material remains unexplored, in much the same way as the manifest content of a dream is discarded in favour of latent dream thoughts.

In summary, the reduced interest in the psychosexual may be due to (a) its close connection with a problematic drive theory, (b) the unconscious resistance and/or conscious prudishness of psychoanalysts, (c) the Kleinian tendency to reduce psychosexuality to the earliest libidinal stages, (d) the increased proportion of psychoanalytic patients with borderline psychopathology for whom sexual interpretations are unhelpful, or (e) the incompatibility of an object-relations theory based on the observation of mother–infant interaction and drive-theory accounts leading to a tendency to reduce sexual material to a presumed underlying relationship-based pathology. In essence, these, and perhaps other changes in psychoanalysis, led to a state of affairs in which sexuality at times appears no more acceptable in the context of a psychoanalytic process than it is in other forms of psychotherapy that do not have Freudian roots: cognitive-behaviour therapy, Rogerian client-centred therapy, and so on. The situation we are faced with is that there is almost no current psychoanalytic theory of psychosexuality. Drive theory can give a compelling and rich account of variations in sexual behaviour and impulses (e.g. of patterns of perversion), but not of sexual desire itself, which is just seen as a biological given. As an explanation of desire, it is tautologous: we feel desire because we have a sexual drive. Treating the whole of psychosexuality as a disguised manifestation of an impersonal sexual drive skirts circularity and is intellectually unsatisfactory. Reducing psychosexuality to an expression of early object relationships, by contrast, desexualizes it altogether. This begs innumerable questions about where the power of sexuality originates.

We believe that sex has left psychoanalysis because psychoanalysis has been unable to provide a strong, intellectually satisfying account of it. What is poorly understood can hardly be successfully used as part of an explanation of something else. To get sex back into psychoanalysis, we have to start with a more persuasive model of normal psychosexual experience.

A brief review of modern psychoanalytic ideas of psychosexuality

The limitations of drive and object-relations theory

Two alternative formulations of psychosexuality highlighted by Greenberg and Mitchell's dichotomy between structural and relational orientations in psychoanalysis have been drive theory and object-relations theory. For Freud, anatomy was destiny (Freud, 1924d). The relationship patterns unfolding with instinctual and ego development were assumed to be driven by the presence or absence of the penis. In addition, there was the linked assumption of the "pleasure principle", which ensured that drive tension would seek relief through discharge in the presence of the object. The stages of libidinal development mapped out the ultimate layeredness of adult sexuality in a way that at times seems to us to have been audaciously reductionistic. In adult sexuality we see the geological strata of a developmental progression from 0 to 4 years of age, where the pinnacle of infantile sexual development, the mastery of the Oedipus complex, is also seen as the template of adult genital sexuality. Blocking or conversion of this developmental path is seen as directly generating sexual dysfunction and deviation as well as a variety of psychological problems through the conversion or displacement of libidinal energy away from genital cathexis.

The alternative formulation, perhaps seen in its purest form in the writings of relational theorists such as Steven Mitchell (2002), sees biology and interpersonal processes as constantly and bidirectionally interacting, with neither having primacy over the other. At the extreme, sex can come to be seen to fulfil merely a social function of intimacy or even just sociability. Instincts become a vehicle for a higher-order process driven by interpersonal experience, both infantile and current. Oedipus comes to be seen as no longer a defining moment of sexuality but, rather, as just one of a range of metaphors and constellations of meaning that could be brought to bear on adult sexuality. Fundamentally, in the relational perspective sexuality has been replaced in psychoanalysis by explanations that focus on the long-term consequences of the vulnerability and dependence of the human infant.

Drive theory is inherently limited because of its circularity and because of its failure to accommodate to the observed variability of sexual practices across cultures. Object-relations theory in its pure form fails to accommodate the unique quality of human sexuality that bridges the relationship between mind and body. A fundamental tenet of classical Freudian theory, implicitly rejected by Klein, is that the mind is rooted in the body, that psychic life is built up out of the mental representation of the physical experiences of infants. Erotic experience remains intensely physical, and the failure to incorporate this aspect or reduce physical arousal to a social construction appears to most to create a distorted and shadowy representation of human sexuality (Budd, 2001).

In between these two extremes are partial formulations where Freud's audacity was diluted through the integration of an interpersonalist perspective. Susan Budd (2001) argues that the distinctively British attitude to sexuality contributed to domesticating Freudian sexuality for Anglo-Saxon consumption. The domestication of psychosexuality actually began with Eric Erikson (1950). For Erikson, orality could be restated as representing the mutuality of the feeding relationship; anality also went beyond the bodily experience and could be seen as entailed in the conflict between holding on and letting go in relation to others as well as within the self. Genitality entailed interpersonal intrusion as well as the potential for exclusion. Throughout Erikson's writings there is a higher-order relational configuration superimposed upon the psychological representation of bodily experience.

The Kleinian revision of sexuality was more subtle, but in the same direction. While throughout her writings (e.g. Klein, Heimann, Isaacs, & Riviere, 1946) Klein retains the language of instincts, in assuming intentionality on the part of infants she implicitly prioritizes thoughts and feelings about the objects as driving physical experience. She believes infants to be born ready to love and wish to possess the feeding object. It is the translation of instincts into feelings (Young, 2001) that shifts the emphasis from a biological drive to a relationship experience. As André Green (1995) pointed out, when Klein places the relationship with the breast at the centre of psychoanalytic theorization, sexuality is ousted from the heart of psychoanalytic thinking. It is retranslated into the language of feeding and nurture rather than ecstasy in mutual enjoyment.

While both Klein and the post-Kleinians retain the Oedipus complex as the cornerstone of sexuality (Britton, Feldman, & O'Shaughnessy, 1989), Fairbairn and the independent object-relations theorists emphasize different aspects of the mother–infant relationship. Given the focus of British object-relations theorists on the real—that is, observed—mother–infant relationship, it was perhaps inevitable that formulations about mothers and infants should be de-eroticized. At the heart of Fairbairn's formulation of sexuality is the notion that aspects of social relating can generate overwhelming affect and may therefore be split off from consciousness. Split-off systems continue to seek expression in current relationships, which in some ways resemble the contexts within which the unconscious fantasies were generated. In the context of the individual sexual life, it is paradoxically the anti-libidinal object that may be of greatest importance. In Stoller's construction of sexuality (Stoller, 1985a) it is hostility that is considered to generate sexual excitement in a relational system that involves hostility, fantasy, and the partial dehumanization of the object. It also entails fantasies of triumph, frustration, and secrecy. A slightly different version of this model is offered by Kernberg (1991a, 1991c), who conceives of sexual excitement as aggression in the service of love. This explains why sexual relationships inevitably entail conflict surrounding intimacy. An alternative compromise formulation comes from those object-relations theorists who consider sexuality to be disturbing because it inevitably entails the kind of vulnerability that triggers split-off memories of the helpless infantile condition, and the sexualization of that vulnerability constitutes a defence against it (Harding, 2001).

Neither drive theory nor object-relations theory in their pure form offered a satisfactory formulation of psychosexuality. Indeed, as we have seen, many of the most successful formulations combine relational and structural theory approaches to arrive at a satisfactory formulation. The work of André Green may be a good example. Green (1997b) allows for a subjective dimension to drives by suggesting that drive is the "*matrix of the subject*" (p. 347) and combines this with the introduction of an impersonal mechanistic character to object relations by replacing the notion of the object, nowadays too readily confused with that of a person, with the "*objectalizing function*". Green (1997a) proposed the idea of "an erotic chain". Drives should not be seen simply as a motivating force contained within the id of the structural model (what French psychoanalysts tend to call "the second topography"). Rather, Green suggests that sexuality unfolds through a series of "formations". These formations are sequenced starting with the dynamic movements of the drive (primary process or defensive distortions), going on to actions that discharge the drive, followed by the experience of pleasure or unpleasure associated with the discharge, and then desire expressed in a state of waiting and search. At this stage, unconscious and conscious representations can feed the desire. A yet further stage of unfolding is the creation of conscious and unconscious fantasies that organize scenarios of wish-fulfilment. Finally, the language of sublimations creates the infinite richness of the erotic and the amorous that defines adult psychosexuality. We have here a chain of signifiers of eroticism that are linked, despite their heterogeneity and different levels of experience and representation, in a reverberating, recurrent sequence. Instead of fixing a certain point in sexuality, the interest is in a dynamic movement in this sequence.

Green's model differs from that of Freud in that it unpacks the process of drive-based mental function into several levels of representational systems or signifiers. He criticizes object-relations theorists and classical drive theorists for attempting to reduce psychosexuality to a single centre of this chain. Thus Kleinians are wrong to equate drives with unconscious fantasy, which is but one of the links within this chain. He implicitly criticizes classical Freudians for focusing exclusively on the beginning of the chain. In his view the appropriate strategy must be to track the chain through its dynamic movements. Psychosexuality is seen as a process that makes use of and is related to the various formations of the psyche (ego, superego, etc.) as well as different kinds of defences. While we do not share Green's views on the specific sequencing, the notion of identifying psychosexuality with the dynamic (developmental) unfolding of a mental process rather than a specific set of static structures, is probably the most effective way of integrating object relational thinking with a drive model.

In conclusion, the problem of relational versus drive tends to be fudged in an "all-deserve-prizes"-type conclusion. Simply put, it is claimed that the gratification of the human sexual drive requires intimacy with another person. Sexuality directed exclusively towards drive gratification is developmentally less advanced than sex that involves love and concern for a partner. Mendoza (cited in Harding, 2001) claims the former type of sexuality, which he terms phallic, to be characteristic of paranoid-schizoid thinking and the latter type, termed genital, to characterize sex in the depressive position. Of course this distinction fails to deal with the possible object-relations roots of sexuality *per se.* It merely states that sexual and relational needs exist side by side, and "mature" sex combines the two in adaptive ways.

The controversies concerning perversion

Freud's definitive statement on sexuality in the *Three Essays on the Theory of Sexuality* (1905d) makes it clear that he viewed human sexuality as basically infinitely variable. Human beings have the capacity to give up the biological function associated with activities such as eating or defecation and hijack it for erotic pleasure. He asserted that bisexuality was ubiquitous and that sexual drives could attach to an almost infinite variety of activities. A person's sexuality was individual, reflecting past histories of gratifications and frustrations, biological predisposition, and current circumstance. Nevertheless, he considered same-sex relationships to violate an underlying biological order that overrode psychological and social considerations. This assumption has been challenged by numerous authors who consider sexuality to be socially constructed and not determined by biology (Giddens, 1992). Giddens regards this as part of the progressive replacement of structures and events that had been external parameters of human activity by socially organized processes. Once sexuality became a part of social relations in place of reproduction, heterosexuality could no longer be the standard by which everything else is judged. This contrasts with Freud's understanding of perversions as the continuation into adulthood of the polymorphous aims and objects of infantile sexuality. In "A Child Is Being Beaten" (1919e), Freud sees perversions as defences against oedipal anxieties, but even this softened, less biologically deterministic approach sits poorly with a social context where the range of socially acceptable sexual practices extends a considerable way beyond genital sex between men and women. This has naturally led to a "normalization" of sexual activities that had previously been considered perversions. Kernberg (1995) for example writes about the potential for couples to deepen their intimacy through full expression of polymorphous sexuality.

A tendency in modern psychoanalytic thinking about psychosexuality is the bringing together of eroticism and perversion (Stein, 1998b). Psychoanalysts who address psychosexual issues commonly claim that, in fantasy at least, there is little to separate normal sexuality from the perversions (Chodorow, 1994; Fogel & Myers, 1991; Kernberg, 1992; McDougall, 1995). A number of different approaches have been proposed to explain this link. For example, McDougall (1995) suggests that the ubiquity of pregenital and primitive internal object relations in psychosexuality might explain this. Kernberg (1992) also points to the symbolic activation of early object relations. The hallmark of this is the splitting of the object and its exploitation even in normal sexual interactions. In his view the splitting heightens the sexual pleasure, bringing the individual closer to oedipal and pre-oedipal object relations. Stoller (1985a) is more specific, seeing the desire to humiliate (and be humiliated) as at the centre of both normal and perverse sexual excitement. What differentiates the non-perverse is the level of intimacy that the individual is capable of achieving with the other, given this emotional context. All sexuality contains hatred, though certain types—such as paedophilia—contain more; what differentiates the non-perverse is the extent to which an erotic act is used for the purpose of avoiding intimacy. In essence all these ideas assert that all sexuality, not just perverted sexuality, springs from the perversion of genital aims (Stein, 1998b). Separating psychosexuality from genitality also seems to us an important aspect of a modern theory of sexuality. For example, Meltzer distinguishes between polymorphous sex and the underlying unconscious fantasies. For example, homosexuality may be healthy or unhealthy (imbued with destructive, aggressive impulses), depending on the underlying unconscious fantasies, as may heterosexuality. Glasser contributed significantly to this controversy in his writings, helping us to understand the connection between aggression and distorted and perverse sexuality. He observed that all of us act aggressively when our mental survival appears at risk. For individuals for whom sexuality poses an existential risk of this kind because of an intense longing for fusion and merger that they experience as part of sexual arousal, an aggressive response of self-defence is understandable. Such individuals erotize the aggression aroused by their merger fantasies and maintain sexual relationships at a safe distance without a fear of annihilation through fusion.

A separate school of thought concerning perversion defines perverse sexuality as an attempt to deceive oneself and others in relation to the basic realities of life, such as oedipal dilemmas. These principally French authors, such as Chasseguet-Smirgel (1985) and Joyce McDougall (1995), assume that in perversion there is a reinvention of the primal scene that denies either the immaturity of the child or the difference between the sexes as the pain associated with these is simply too much to bear.

In summary, within most modern psychoanalytic formulations the almost infinite variety of sexuality is accepted as normal and bounded only by the human imagination. However, like any human activity, sexuality is seen as serving multiple functions, and it is the service to which sexuality is put that indicates a fundamentally maladaptive character. Thus sexuality in the service of psychic survival, the substitution of a pseudo-relatedness for genuine intimacy, the disguising of hostility or hatred, or the erotization of aggression that could be triggered by intimacy—in these contexts modern psychoanalysis considers sexuality to be perverse. The key indicators are not the fantasy nor the activity but, rather, the compulsive, restrictive, and anxiety-driven character. Normality and perversion is thus an inappropriate dimension that could and should be replaced by our understanding of the degree to which a particular type of sexual activity serves functions other than erotic pleasure.

Sexuality and the analytic relationship

Transference was, of course, where the psychoanalytic view of sexuality started. Confronted with the puzzle of how an attractive young woman (Anna O) could fall in love with an ugly middle-aged man (Dr Breuer), Freud's genius hit upon the concept of transference and, within that category of experiences, erotic transferences that could be traced back to childhood sexuality in general and oedipal experiences in particular. The repressed erotic feelings towards the parent of the opposite gender were considered by Freud to be reactivated by the therapeutic relationship. It was not until much later that Freud realized that intense sexual experiences within the analysis indicated an incapacity to think about the nature of these experiences and in preference to analytic reflection to re-experience and enact. As the mother–infant model replaced the oedipal model as the prototypical template of transference, erotic transference was increasingly seen as originating not in the Oedipus complex but, rather, in failures at earlier stages of reality. Mann (1997), for example, suggested that the erotization of the transference was rooted in a regression to a primitive confusional state where experiences are not clearly located as firmly in either the child or the mother. The suggestion here is similar to that of Laplanche (see below), suggesting that the threat of maternal sexuality to the infant to use the infant to satisfy her own sexual need is "transferred" to the therapeutic relationship. This leads to a defensive de-erotization of the therapeutic relationship.

The relational perspective adds a twist and complexity to this already controversial theme. Harold Searles (1959) makes a convincing case that for the analysis to work, the analyst needs to actually fall in love with the patient. The curative power of the "real relationship" between patient and analyst is highlighted by orthodox clinicians such as Loewald (1960) and perhaps more controversially by Winnicott (1972). However, the relational perspective suggested by authors such as Ehrenberg (1993), Pizer (1998), and Hoffman (1998) creates a particular challenge. If the analyst's sexual feelings are considered inevitably to penetrate his relationship with the patient, given the myth of analytic neutrality and the theoretical and to some degree practical deconstruction of analytic boundaries, the intensification of sexuality in the context of a therapeutic relationship, combined with the focus on the real relationship, creates a situation of grave risk for the violation of boundaries. It is hardly surprising that analysts have traditionally found a way of blaming their patient for their vulnerability in this context. Freud wrote to Jung: "*The way these women manage to charm us with every conceivable psychic perfection until they have attained their purpose is one of nature's greatest spectacles*".

Technical innovations from self-psychologists, interpersonalist-relational therapists, intersubjectivists, and classical analysts embracing notions such as role-responsiveness (Sandler, 1976) or the "total transference" (Joseph, 1985) have challenged us further as to delineating the "proper boundaries" of analytic technique. This chapter does not deal with the rights and wrongs of such changes of legitimate therapeutic style. Such questions are mistakenly classed with ethical conundrums. They firmly belong in the domain of empiricism. The ethical stance is to work in the manner that has been shown to be most likely to help our patients. My concern here is with understanding unequivocally iniquitous conduct. Boundary "crossings" implied by technical innovations are probably harmless and perhaps effective components of long-term therapy (Glass, 2003; Gutheil & Gabbard, 1993), but boundary violations involve serious and deleterious misconduct. Both probably arise out of enactments of unconscious phantasies activated in the participants of the therapeutic relationship, but the former requires systematic study in terms of evaluations of the impact of modification of therapeutic style on outcome, while the latter calls for scrutiny of the process of its genesis with a view to its prevention and comprehensive eradication.

Developmental views of psychosexuality

A further current perspective, somewhat different from classical formulations on sexuality, is offered by Laplanche's comprehensively elaborated theory (Fletcher, 1992; Laplanche, 1995; Laplanche & Pontalis, 1968), which we will brutally reduce to four propositions.

(1) Laplanche claims that psychosexuality evolves in infancy out of non-sexual, instinctual activity. When the non-sexual instinct, having generated excitation, *loses* its natural object, the ego is turned upon itself and is left in a state of arousal. Laplanche terms this arousal "an auto-erotic moment" that comes to be elaborated through perception and fantasy in what he calls "phantasmatization". The replacement of the object by a fantasy lies, for Laplanche, at the root of psychosexuality.

(2) This sense of autoerotic excitement is not objectless, but, importantly, its object is an *internal state*: the desire is for the idea of the lost object, and presumably all the internal states that accompany the experience of loss in the moment of excitement. This also means that even if the object that is lost is the breast, it can never be found, because what is desired is no longer the actual feeding breast but the "phantasmatic" breast, the breast elaborated through fantasy. This is what gives human sexual experience its essentially non-functional character. (This is an intellectually far more satisfactory account than the essentially circular claim that human sexuality is instinctual—that is, self-preservative—except that it happens to be more or less permanently activated.) It is also at the root of the object-seeking character that completely permeates normal human sexuality.

(3) Combining these two ideas, a model of sexuality emerges in which bodily arousal has become sexualized. But this psychosexual need, unlike a sexual instinct, can never be satisfied because its object is inherently unattainable. It is ultimately impossible to rediscover the object, as the lost object is "phantasmatic" and the found object has to be real. However, Laplanche recognized that this formulation

begs the question of why instinctually generated excitement should be so powerfully channelled towards the sexual. The profound contribution he makes is introducing the idea of the sexualization of the infant's arousal by the mother. This has been partially recognized by a number of other psychoanalytic authors (Lichtenstein, 1977; Spitz, 1945), including Freud (1910c). Ultimately it is the mother's unconscious "seduction" of the infant, claims Laplanche, that converts instinctual excitement to the autoerotic moment.

(4) Laplanche considers that the infant is not ready to integrate this experience with other experiences of the mother. This could be because of the dynamically unconscious nature of the interaction, which leaves the infant with sense of inaccessible meaning, or what Laplanche calls enigma. It is incontrovertible that erotic experience is imbued with mystery (Kernberg, 1992; Stoller, 1985a). The mystery may be rooted in the enigmatic quality of the mother's gestures, which initially colours the infant's experience of his excitement but then serves to intensify the seduction, finally becoming its central feature. Ruth Stein (1998a), in an inspiring review of Laplanche's work, actually makes this explicit: "the primal enigma shapes the sexual object relationship, and is later expressed by it" (p. 605). Two aspects of this process—the lost object found and the uncovering of an enigma—are seen in the intensely erotic quality of hiding and revealing sexual areas of the body, even in cultures where near-nakedness is normal.

Attractive as these ideas are intellectually, they fall short of a full explanation of sexuality. In particular, it is not clear exactly how the experience of frustration can come to be desirable through maternal seduction. Further, the nature of this "seduction", while evocative of the intimacy of the mother–infant relationship and thus intellectually quite appealing, remains vague and somewhat improbable. There is little room in the theory for interpersonal relationships that undoubtedly shape adult sexuality. Our purpose here is not to criticize Laplanche's model but, rather, to build on these powerful ideas, keeping in mind recent suggestions concerning the development of the agentive self (Fonagy & Target, submitted).

At the heart of Laplanche's idea is the claim that the driven quality of human psychosexuality is not a property of the sexual drive but derives from the need to pursue a lost object that has become imaginary (phantasmatic) and is displaced from the original functional loss. There seem to us to be two major areas in which the theory

Laplanche has developed could be made even more compelling using developmental elaborations: the first is to elaborate the basic mechanism involved in the sexualization of non-instinctual tension through the mother's seductiveness, and the second is to address how object-finding and object relations become the principal expression of normal psychosexuality in adulthood. The first of these two aspects is related to the process of mirroring that underpins the infant becoming aware of mental states (Gergely & Watson, 1996), while the second is the unfolding of the unassimilated (enigmatic) *Anlage* of this mirroring process in adult relationships. What makes this integration of ideas particularly poignant are the self-evident similarities between the phenomenology of borderline states and normal sexuality.

Sexual excitement *per se* has complex developmental links with the emergence of subjectivity. In an as yet unpublished paper, Mary Target and I (Fonagy & Target, submitted) have advanced an attachment theory approach to the understanding of human sexuality based largely on our model of the development of affect representation outlined above. In summary, we have suggested that emotions associated with sexual arousal in the infant are never accurately mirrored by the mother because of her appropriate unconscious respect for the infant's person boundaries. The infant's high drive state may become sexualized if the mother becomes excited by the baby's arousal and momentarily breaks her contact with the baby, who thus loses its object and sexualizes the mother's excited turning away, internalizing an excited, alienated presence. A specific quality of this excitement is that while it is experienced as within, its incongruence with the infant's actual experience disrupts the coherence of the self. A key facet of psychosexuality, then, is a sense of incongruence in relation to the experience of the self. It can never truly be experienced as owned. What Freud (1905d) talked about as an objectless state and Laplanche (1995) and Ruth Stein (1998a) as the "enigmatic other", we describe in terms of an "alien part of the self" internalized by the alienating parts of the mirroring object–mother. The infant takes the mother's displays to be mirroring his own experience and thus identifies them as his own, yet since they are not mirrored "contingently" (that is, in a manner faithful to his own affects and experiences), they are also experienced as not his own at the same time. The internalization of a distracting and seductive response to frustration gives the psychosexual core its unique combination of urgency and playfulness. The enigmatic dimension of sexuality creates an invitation that calls out to be elaborated, normally by an other.

Normal sexual excitement is by nature incongruent with the self, and it has therefore to be experienced in the other and as a consequence with the other. When one distances oneself significantly from one's partner's mind state, there is little chance that one will be sexually excited by them. In the analytic setting the analyst's concern with the enigmatic is inevitably sexually stimulating. I can think of only two categories of interpersonal interaction where the exchange of subjectivities across a person's physical boundaries is both mutually desired and legitimized: one is normal sexual excitement, and the other is psychoanalysis. The intersubjective exchange between patient and analyst creates a setting where the sexual self is placed in the physically proximal other to reduce incongruity. It is projected into and observed in the other and enjoyed since normal sexual excitement is always felt to be the experience of the other rather than of the self. Since the true pleasure of erotism derives from the opportunity to transpose oneself into a state of mind that is felt to be the other's, there will always be something inherently sexualized even in the routine non-sexual intersubjective processes that psychoanalysis entails. Psychosexuality is the internalization of a misreading, an attempt to grasp something that is excessive, asymmetrical, and strange. Sex can never be fully experienced alone, because it is only through the projection of the alien part of the self into the other and seeing it there that the individual can make full contact with their true constitutional self state of excitement. It is therefore, in my view, inevitable that any situation where the "enigmatic" is activated will also arouse sexual excitement. It is the reinternalization of the other's excitement through identification that consolidates the intersubjective bond.

Because normal sexuality depends on the demolition of intersubjective boundaries and the abolishing of the limitations of one's separate existence, it follows that psychoanalysis as an activity (not as a therapeutic process) mimics by analogy the mechanisms that underpin sexual excitement. In particular, it will be therapeutic relationships where the therapist shares some aspects of the subjective experience of the patient that are likely to elicit a response of sexual excitement from the patient. Similarly, the therapist's efforts to enliven the patient, to create a safe and secure intersubjective domain, will create an unusual opportunity for him to experience his excitement through the patient's subjectivity, to which he is so closely linked. Given the structural similarities of psychoanalytic therapy and the nature of sexual excitement, what might surprise us is the relative infrequency with which sexual boundary violations occur rather than their disturbingly high prevalence. It is a testament to the method invented by Freud, which has its focus on clarifying the distinctions between self and other states, that sexual boundary violations do not occur more often.

SUMMARY AND CONCLUSION

We have started this brief review by noting that sexuality has, to some extent, left psychoanalysis. This is clearly inappropriate in the light of our increased awareness of the importance of biology for the study of the mind. At a time when cognitive psychologists are moving increasingly towards the body in their attempts to understand complex mental structures, it would be a shame if the profession that was one of the first to focus on the bodily origins of mental processes were to shy away from the importance of sexuality in our mental functioning. Sex has undoubtedly become more complex since Freud's original descriptions, yet in another way it has changed little. It is still there as the primary motor ensuring the survival of our species, the perpetuation of our genetic material. For all mammals the process of reproduction is at the centre of their behavioural systems. For mammals with minds, this is unlikely to be different. Sexual inhibition and dissatisfaction, conflicts and perversions, the sheer intensity of guilt, jealousy, and rage that sexuality entails, are indicators of how central sexual function remains for us. Psychoanalysis cannot shirk its traditional responsibility of casting light into the darkest recesses of our mental existence.

2

Sexuality: a conceptual and historical essay

André E. Haynal

Some historical hints

Sexuality has been at the centre of interest of psychoanalysis. Is it still today? What was the *novelty* Freud brought into this domain? There is no doubt that sexuality was also at the centre of Freud's interest. He used bits and pieces of the then new observations and the discourse of the contemporary sexologists to lay the foundation for his own new science. But what were the news he put before the eyes of a stunned world of 1905, a century ago, provoking much admiration and much resistance?

First let us remember that at the time of the publication of *The Interpretation of Dreams* (1900a), he wrote to Fliess: "A theory of sexuality might well be the dream book's immediate successor" and its complement (1905d, p. 129, Letter 128). Why this? We may speculate that discovering the sexual nature and the unconscious *wish* at the root of the dreams led him more than other former experiences with sexuality to the elaboration of its theory. The instinctual drives became the foundation of *fantasy life,* and this has remained perhaps the most important element in psychoanalytic practice until today. It is perhaps no coincidence that he always tried to keep these two books, the one on dreams and that on sexuality—and only these—up to date. They were the pillars of his doctrine.

In general terms, on the cultural scene, he allowed people to *speak* about sexuality. The author of the *Aphasia Studies* created a language and, together with others such as Krafft-Ebing, supplied terms like masochism, sadism, narcissism, inhibition, and many others, allowing what one thought about sex to be formulated. He brought the sexually determined contents out of the closet of medical consultation-room and the Latin jargon into everyday language. In a little circle of men—who also had some sexual problems of their own, as in the case of Stekel, Ferenczi, Jones, Tausk, Gross, Jung, and others—the sensitivity for this dimension was brought to life so that a scientific discourse could slowly emerge, partly borrowed from the sexologists.

Moreover, if Freud considered that Iwan Bloch's merits consisted in having replaced "the pathological approach" of homosexuality with "the anthropological one" (1905d, p. 139, n. 2), he simultaneously named the direction in which himself would go. Yes, "anthropological" is the word Freud uses, in spite of his reserves against philosophy: in fact, a new *anthropology* was born, of human beings seen as profoundly rooted in nature and, among other things, in their instinctual heritage.

When there are cracks in a building, there are two possibilities: one can either fill them in and try to repair the damage or tear the building down and build a new one. The latter way is exactly how Freud handled turn-of-the-century sexology, and the new building that emerged was called *psychoanalysis*. In other words, we can say that in 1905, sexology and psychoanalysis entered into some kind of (short-lived) marriage. The first part of the *Three Essays on the Theory of Sexuality* quotes practically all of the authors of the then newly emerging science of sex (1905d, p. 135), beginning with Freud's well-known friend Wilhelm Fliess; even later, he always kept an eye on the contributions about biology and endocrinology (1920g, p. 60; 1933a, p. 182; 1916–17, pp. 389, 414ff). This importance is also expressed in his complaint at the very end of the *Three Essays*: "We know far too little of the biological processes constituting the essence of sexuality to be able to *construct* from our *fragmentary* information a theory" (1905d, p. 243; italics added).

It was also new that Freud came to conceive of human sexuality as situated in a *continuum* that starts at the very beginning of life, implying that adult sexuality, in its mature form, was to be seen as an accomplishment in a developmental process. If "sex is fun", Freud told us, in any fun and pleasure there is some sex. Moreover, he further stressed its importance in considering remnants of sexual excitements or inhibitions as building block of the *personality* structure. Consequently, sexuality came to be considered as the foundation for our *relationships* with others, be they more or less intimate, and as forcefully contributing to our social framework, according to the attraction or repulsion between individuals. All this gave occasion for his scientific opponents to accuse him of "pansexualism", which, seen in this sense, might have been justified to some extent. (We can add that, in their wake, modern ethologists tend to see a similar infiltration, if not inundation, of sexuality also in everyday interactions of other primates, as, for example, in certain chimpanzees called bonobos—Schäppi, 1998.)

This topic never ceased to occupy Freud. On the contrary: it led him to new bits of understanding, up to the exploration of the masochistic fantasies of his own daughter (Freud, 1924c), and it affected his understanding of most of his clinical cases.

Maybe we should read Freud differently from the customary way of studying him: instead of looking into his work for facts and truths as presented in the usual way of the natural sciences and also in the medical model, why don't we rather look out for and be rewarded with *stimulations*, with visions. He told us himself that "I do not wish to arouse conviction; I wish to stimulate thought and to upset prejudices." (1916–17, p. 243).

As a matter of fact, the impact of his thoughts on the *popular culture* of the twentieth century, including a sometimes simplistic use of its terminology that has invaded our language, has often been brought to our attention. Films, theatre, and books like the works of James Joyce, Virginia Woolf, or of the French surrealists are unimaginable without Freud's contributions to culture, even if the way they later borrowed his ideas was not always along the lines of the intentions of the originator, the Master. For Freud: "Where id was, there ego shall be"—and this was not always understood by these authors in its dimension of taking up a project that ultimately goes back to Goethe, Schopenhauer, and Nietzsche. The ego, the individual, should in Freud's intentions realize his/her full potential, his/her self—an aim that became influential above all in our culture of the second half of the twentieth century.

Heritage

Beyond the impact on popular culture, however, we have to ask ourselves whether *psychoanalysis itself* has been true to this heritage, or whether it has abandoned it. A sensitive question, all the more so in view of Freud's constant evolution regarding this topic. Let us remind ourselves that the important concepts on *infantile sexuality* and on the *pregenital* organization of the libido made their appearance as late as 1905 (1905d, p. 126). It is only then that it could be clarified how partial drives become "condensed into one complex buzz" in genitality (Stoller, 1979b, p. 26). Now the relation between adolescent and adult sexuality becomes clear, whereas before there was "no doubt a confusion between sexual and genital" (Freud, 1905d, 180).

Along the same line of reasoning, he declared that the "same disposition to perversions of every kind is a general and fundamental human characteristic" (1905d, 191). Normal sexual behaviour develops out of this disposition (1905d, p. 231). Even if, as Sulloway (1979) showed, Freud took a great many of his ideas from Fliess, particularly from his friend's book of 1897, he elaborated the topic in a new perspective: that of concentrating on and clarifying the person's inner world.

In a similar vein, Freud wrote on "sexual aberrations" (1905d, p. 135) and immediately called for a re-evaluation in showing that we are able to *understand*, instead of simply dismiss, what comes to us under the label of aberration.

In this constant evolution, there already appear the first hints of concepts that were more fully elaborated only much later, either by Freud himself or by other psychoanalysts. Upon close reading, we already find the notion of the "*grasping instinct*", which manifests "itself . . . [in] catching hold of some part of another person" (1905d, p. 180)—a precursor of the later concept of *clinging* and, still later, perhaps that of *attachment*.

Likewise, from 1905 onwards the *libido* is theoretically presented as an endogenous energy that unfolds in a preordained developmental path. The theory is based on the supposition that a vital function—for example, the ingestion of food—gives such pleasure that, as a consequence, this pleasure and the seeking of pleasure become detached from the primary biological goal: "satisfaction . . . becomes detached from the need for taking nourishment" (1905d, p. 182).

Freud called those distinct areas, which are most important for this pleasure-seeking, "erotogenic zones", but in fact the entire surface of our skin comes to be considered an erotogenic zone (p. 182): our whole body can become erotogenic when fuelled by appropriate fantasies. The wish for the presence of others, for closeness, intimacy, attachment, and detachment-separation can (later) be situated in this dimension.

Many of these remarks by Freud mark the beginnings of the lines of a "post-Freudian evolution". Thus, in his wake, the exploration of *pregenital* pleasures or of the *narcissistic* dimension have become major topics for several authors. By defining sexuality in a broad way, Freud seems to have opened the door to an advance in such a direction, in an evolution in which he himself took an active part.

It is interesting to note, moreover, that he did not do away with, but continued to use, the *observational* method of his forerunners: the second of the *Three Essays,* on "The Infantile Sexuality", is in reality a psychoanalytic observational study. It is true that he did not make systematic studies of his own, as he complains to Fliess that the "womenfolk do not support my researches and did not appreciate my going into the nursery and experiment with Annerl" (E. Freud, 1960, p. 230). This is interesting as the legitimacy of such an observational method has recently been doubted (see Sandler, Green, & Stern, 2000) under the lingering influence of Lacan, in spite of Freud's preference for the "co-operation of the two methods" (1905d, p. 201).

In general, in my view, the later *evolution* of ideas does not seem to stand in opposition to the seeds Freud sowed. As I see it, it is only the concentration on the *defence mechanisms* in analysis, *instead of* on the sexually centred contents, that has caused something of a shift away from the understanding of the underlying sexual material that pervades the psychoanalytic situation (as well as life in general). This intellectualization and "*obsessionalization*" of the psychoanalytic technique has sometimes led to a "drying out" of its dynamics and an incapability to create links between various elements that constitute the analytic discourse. This prevents any possibility of creative encounters with drives stemming from hitherto unexplored depths, positive sources of the authentic personality, the real self. One may even wonder whether this evolution did not play its role, in some regions of the world, in the fading interest in psychoanalysis, which has more and more come to be considered as boring.

Another danger of neglecting the sexual dimension is that it may lead to an exclusively *phenomenological* understanding of the discourse of the analysand, which deprives psychoanalysis of an important dimension in understanding his or her personality.

Some critics, even from the Freudian camp, seem to forget the extension of this concept. The complaint that there is less sexual material in today's clinical presentations than was the case before may perhaps be justified with regard to the most elaborate layers of adult sexuality—in other words, actual genital activity—but it has to be qualified if we do not limit this notion of sexuality to genitality. (As in the case of my 18-year-old patient, whose excitement and pleasure in driving his father's car is certainly linked to pleasures of competition, of mastery, and perhaps even to pregenital vertigo. In connection with these fantasies we find an oedipal constellation, even with a pleasure-giving, admired maternal figure.) Sometimes the same persons who consider themselves Freudians forget how the libido is silently working behind the scenes, in the unconscious, and can only be grasped indirectly. These forces are concealed, but nevertheless give psychoanalytic listening a specific flavour. If this is forgotten, we end up in pure phenomenology, far removed from the Freudian reference system that has shown over the course of a century how subtly these fantasies are always present.

Fantasy

In contemporary clinical psychoanalysis, the important aspect of sexuality is still the leading force behind our fantasies (see King & Steiner, 1991) and, as such, remains a prevalent expression of wishes and desires. Even if working with underlying sexual fantasies in the psychoanalytic situation has, historically speaking, taken different forms, its central role has never been disputed, whether we proceed with the method of a *direct translation* on an oro-genital level like Melanie Klein in her account of Richard (Klein, 1961) or with more indirect methods.

Freud himself, from the beginning, thought of *separation* and the ensuing absence of the other as important factors having an impact on fantasy life. We read, for example: "he was afraid of . . . the absence of someone he loved; and he could feel sure of being soothed as soon as he had evidence of that person's presence" (1905d, p. 224, n.1). A main feature of tenderness arising from the secure presence is especially important in the mother–child relationship.

This is important not only for the child, but also in old age, as Graham Greene, a great *connoisseur* of human sexual life, writes in his beautiful prose: "At the end of what is called 'the sexual life' the only love which has lasted is the love that has accepted everything, every disappointment, every failure and every betrayal, which has accepted even the sad fact that in the end there is no desire so deep as the simple desire for companionship" (Graham Greene, *"May We Borrow Your Husband?"*). Even Erik H. Erikson, in his conception of human tasks at different ages, would agree to see tenderness being integrated in this way into the stage of *maturity*. In any case, it seems that this is what he has been living through . . .

Again and again, in an infinite evolution, we can discover new ways of understanding classical themes and scenes, as in fantasies of the primal scene where parental sex takes place behind closed doors—where the child finds him- or herself *excluded*. This can mobilize feelings of humiliation, inadequacy, or rejection and may help also to form an impression that what is closed, unacceptable, forbidden becomes the really exciting thing. This is also one of the cases when a fear is ultimately converted into pleasure—one might say, "resexualized" (Person, 1995: 82). If the unavailable and unattainable partner has more aphrodisiac power than a sexual partner lying in our bed, it has something to do with the attraction of the forbidden. Thus, without doubt, fantasies determine important aspects of life. Moreover, they can be a compass for the choices we make with regard to the future (Sandler).

In our analyses, we can also understand certain aspects of what is called "*real life*". For example, the term "pornography" derives etymologically from the Greek *porné*, prostitute, and the verb *graphein*, to describe. The pornographer deals, in the first place, with matters of prostitution, and only in modern usage does the connotation encompass any graphic portrayal of sexuality. The price to pay for the voyeuristic pleasure and the exhibition of the other certainly includes an element of humiliation. This is in the line of thinking of the late Robert Stoller, who qualified hostility as the driving force in desire and excitement. "The hostility of eroticism is an attempt, repeated over and over, to undo childhood traumas and frustrations" (Stoller, 1979b, p. 6). If one of the functions of dreams is to overcome traumatic elements activated by daily events, it may also be the element of *"bonification"*—a tendency to restore the psychic balance—that plays a similarly important role in sexuality. (Theoretically this means that behind sexuality there is not only libido, but also *destrudo.*)

Speaking about fantasies of humiliation derived from the aggressive drive, we find these again in fantasies or enactments of coprolalia or urethral activity or other practices, such as bondage, that lead us *directly* to humiliation itself, to masochism, and to the death drive.

The complexity of sexual fantasies behind a given sexual behaviour does not allow a one-to-one translation between them. This great complexity underlies actual sexual behaviour, and it is no coincidence that certain psychoanalysts such as Robert Stoller, more interested in studying this complexity, could even go as far as saying that psychoanalysts do not know sexual behaviour—that is, what people actually do in their sexual activities.

The examination of *culture* teaches us much about sexuality. Freud and the Freudians showed, roughly in opposition to the sexologists, that sexuality and gender are not products of nature alone, but are also moulded by experience. In formulating the dimension of sexuality and desire with reference to its *relational side*, we have to bear in mind the fact that sexuality entails an interpenetration of bodies and needs, and it makes its endless variations ideally suited to represent longings, conflicts, and negotiations in the relations between self and others. Sex is a powerful organizer of experience. Bodily sensations and sensual pleasures define one's skin, one's outline, one's boundaries; and the dialectics of bodily and sexual intimacies position one in relation to the other: over, under, inside, against, surrounding, controlling, yielding, adored, enraptured, and so on.

> The powerful biological surges in the phenomenology of sexual excitement, the sense of being "driven", provide a natural vocabulary for dramatic expression of dynamics involving conflict, anxiety, compulsion, escape, passion, and rapture [Mitchell, 1988, p. 103]

Freud drew from his experiences, and the evolution of his thoughts was constantly in movement, as we can see best in that parallel "logbook" that is his vast correspondence. In his evolution, the *cultural and social context* certainly also played a role. We can measure the impact of the *Zeitgeist* when we compare the Freud (1912f) of the discussions on masturbation, expressing negative opinions and uncertainties, with the view of a contemporary psychoanalyst: "Masturbation is also powerful because it provides an independent and autonomous source of satisfaction; we are no longer entirely dependent on another person to fulfil our needs and desires" (Person, 1995, p. 82).

Gender theory and couvade

It would be interesting to go into Freud's gender theory and the subsequent discussions with Jones and the female psychoanalysts in his environment—an important topic, until now, of discussion under the headline of "female sexuality" (1920a, 1925j, 1931b, 1933a), but the limitations of space do not allow this. I would rather take up a problem of gender identity in men during the pregnancy of their wives and the childbirth. A patient, in whom delusions were triggered by these events, led me to discover that various rituals, called *couvade*, accompany these events in many cultures—until recently even in Europe, in the Basque country and in some regions of France. Their aim is the consolidation of masculine identity based on bisexuality tied to difficult problems of rivalry, uncertainty about paternity, and other fantasies connected with these. Freud (1908c, pp. 223–224) once mentioned this anthropological fact, and one of his close and valued collaborators (Reik, 1914) wrote a study about it (see also Haynal, 1968, 1977). My good fortune may be that during a stay in Malaysia I was able to observe this custom myself. I realized that we are perhaps not sufficiently attentive to similar problems in our patients. The high rate of divorce after childbirth may also be linked to this complex problem around this biological—and *not only* biological—event.

Seduction

I would like to say a few words here about problems that are, in my view, fundamental in human life from its beginning (see also Laplanche, 1988, 1995), and also in psychoanalysis, and are, perhaps, not always sufficiently valued: seduction as an example of the presence of *sexuality* in everyday life.

Seduction can be defined as an active movement of establishing contact, or a growing *intimacy*. Establishing contact means mobilization of *libido*. This complex affective phenomenon is frequently communicated by emotional, non-verbal channels, such as looks, gestures, voice, posture, and so forth. The setting-up of an analytic bond, and thus of the *process* of analysis, takes place by setting in motion a movement of mutual seduction. As many channels of affective communication via visual signs are blocked in analysis, it is the analyst's offer of a presence, an intense listening, his honesty, his expectations, and his demands that carry the seductive message. In this *perspective*—Bion's "vertex" (1965, pp. 106–107)—we are able to grasp the affective emotional set-up of the process. Remember that in his earlier works, Freud's preoccupations revolve around problems of seduction and sexuality, raised by the encounters with his analysands; these became the starting point of the adventure he came to call psychoanalytic treatment.

To begin with the analyst's seduction: what greater seduction is there than to offer to listen, attentively, four or five times a week, and thus become, on a regular basis, the centre of interest for the Other—who knows about failed seductions, and how these failures can become traumatic? It is a creation of an affective bond, followed by a "honeymoon", as Béla Grunberger (1971) called it, together with the growing awareness of one's wishes and hopes, and also the fears, anxieties, and profound concerns aroused in both protagonists. It is quite clear that a focus on the *libidinal encounter* and on what it mobilizes will lead to a conception of psychoanalysis in which the *experiencing* of that emotionality and its eventual analysis will play an important role. Denying the role that certain sexual and emotional factors play in it would, at the same time, deprive analysis of understanding a very important dimension of this bonding, taking place in the triangle of sexuality, fantasy, and emotional *experience*.

Libido is responsible for the bonding between persons, as opposed to the death instinct, which causes repulsion, distance, and hostility. It works from the first moment of life, in the creation of the bond between the mother and her child. The mother offers warmth and mutual gaze, touch and milk, and the baby responds with mimicking, warbling, and other vocal manifestations. Its role in everyday life cannot be exaggerated, creating sympathy, attraction, as well as hostility. In the history of psychoanalysis this concept has been overshadowed by the problems of a gross sexual *seduction* in childhood and its pathogenetic role. A rehabilitation of this fine libidinal force in psychoanalysis seems important.

About cases

In some clinical cases, we find a continuity between the subject's basic fantasies and his sexual imaginations. "Marcel", a young man with a very masochistic self-representation and with a life story full of ordeals, re-stages sequences of pain and consolation in his sexual encounters. It is his partner who plays the active role—her hands, her mouth—while Marcel can stay in passive expectation and quasi-total inactivity. He is an impressive example that illustrates the complexity of libidinal fantasies, linked to infantile relations and their failure, hidden behind the sexual behaviour of the adult.

Another man presents an extreme Don Juan syndrome. The deepest source of his behaviour is the fear of being left alone. He cannot bear sleeping alone for *one single* night, out of fear of being abandoned and rejected and having to confront the extreme danger of solitude: an archaic problem, presenting itself with an excessively compelling force. The desire for a maternal presence and its derivative in the always-available woman (Person, 1995), as opposed to this man's experience of the unavailability of certain sexual objects and his dread of rejection by females, seems the principal motivating force. In my opinion this case illustrates well the archaic pregenital problem and its impact on later sexual behaviour.

CONCLUSION

Sexuality, which lies behind fantasies loaded with desire, is at the centre of psychoanalytic work. Moreover, we find no exact correspondence between fantasies and behaviour, as sexual excitement and behaviour are based upon a complexity of genital and pregenital fantasies.

We could say, in paraphrasing Proust: We are always "*à la recherche du fantasme perdu*", searching for lost fantasy, and not simply reading it directly, or easily recognizing sexuality in terms of it.

To sum up: In Freud's thinking and in that of the early pioneers, the notion of sexuality encompassed a complex continuum, involving pregenitality and narcissism. The preoccupation with these dimensions could have given rise to the impression that sexuality has become less important in the contemporary psychoanalytic field. However, if we accept Freud's broad definition of it, we will see that in contemporary psychoanalysis sexuality is also present behind the notions of desire and fantasy. Could it be that here also, as we say in French: *"Plus ça change, plus c'est la même chose"* [The more it changes, the more it stays the same]?

Commentary

Sverre Varvin

André Haynal's chapter is rich, and it is a challenge for thought, reflection, and, I suppose, disagreement. It is stimulating in an almost sensual way, as all threads of thought he picks up from the *Three Essays on the Theory of Sexuality* (1905d) and beyond work as excitations that get our thoughts going. It is rightly in the spirit of Freud, whom he quite appropriately cites: "I do not wish to arouse conviction, I wish to stimulate thought and to upset prejudices" (1916–17, p. 243). It is a work that deserves several readings—readings that may both deepen understanding and also give opportunity to find something new and thought-provoking.

When Haynal states at the end: *"Plus ça change, plus c'est la même chose"* [The more it changes, the more it stays the same], this may be described as the underlying programme of his chapter. After all, when we accept Freud's broad definition of sexuality, we are Freudian, in the sense that what we do as psychoanalysts will always relate to sexuality—or, put another way, revisions of these bases of psychoanalysis, sexuality and the drives, are not easily accomplished and, when tried, they are often not significantly successful. We will always find it fruitful to return to Freud.

André Haynal sharpens the point when he states that sexuality is the link to the innermost of the personality, to the real self; and he claims, further, that the lack of this perspective may be the source, in many places, to the fading interest in psychoanalysis—an important point not taken up in the present discussion on the crisis in psychoanalysis.

So we are faced with a problem: are we in danger of forgetting the basis of psychoanalysis: that infantile sexuality determines human nature, development, and character, and that, whether we are aware of it or not, sexuality or autoerotism pervades the analytic setting? And since this is said in a research context, one could also ask whether the possible impoverished understanding of sexuality and the drives is reinforced by scrutinizing research into the analytic situation, that this activity, necessary as it is, is another example of the "*obsessionalization*" that, according to Haynal, may characterize present-day psychoanalytic technique?

Does this watering-down of psychoanalysis make it just as attractive as any cognitive approach—which, by the way, presents a more straightforward theory for research, as well as for psychotherapeutic education?

Freud managed, especially with the *Three Essays*, to create a new anthropology where man is rooted in nature and in the drives or instincts, but where sexuality is also understood as developing in relationships, which shape them and which, in turn, shape the personality. It is appropriate here to remind ourselves of the distinction, which is not always clear in Haynal's chapter, between instinct and drive ("*Instinkt*" and "*Trieb*" in German). The unfortunate conflation of instinct and drive in the English translation of Freud has confused matters and is at the basis of misunderstandings of the place of sexuality in development: that man is rooted in nature but that this nature becomes culture through the shaping of sexuality and drives in the developmental process. While instinct is more-or-less fixed and geared to adaptation, as Laplanche rightly points out (Laplanche, 2001), drives are non-adaptive, and, even if they have a biological basis, they emerge in the child's relation to the adult and start a process in the child, an autoerotic "reworking", which forms the basis of fantasy, leading eventually to maturity or pathology. Freud suggested, as we know, that the drive or "*Trieb*" is, in itself, without quality but is "so far as mental life is concerned, . . . only to be regarded as a measure of demand made upon the mind for work" (1905d, p. 83).

This work can only be done in a relationship—hence anthropology, as Haynal underlines.

Drives can, accordingly, not be understood in a simple tension-discharge model; they are not aiming at equilibrium. Freud later coined the terms Eros and libido for the binding forces that act as driving force in the psyche, subsuming partial drives under the hegemony of a relation to a whole object. But we are constantly reminded that autoerotism and partial drives are there all the time, as Haynal demonstrates, among others, in the clinical situations described in the vignettes at the end of his chapter.

I focus on the following themes related to Haynal's chapter:

- the relation between drives/instinct and object relations/attachment, primary love
- seduction
- fantasy
- gender
- development
- implications for research

The relation between drives/instinct and object relations/attachment/primary love

It appears to be widely accepted in psychoanalysis today that there is some kind of primary need for relationships, which some claim to be a constitutional predisposition, described variously as, for example, primary love (Balint, 1965), object seeking (Fairbairn, 1952), or ego relatedness (Winnicott, 1960). This is an old debate where modern attachment theory has revitalized the debate with underpinnings from research findings, but surely one that has also contributed to a widening of the gap between drive theory and developmental theories (Fonagy, 2001).

The drive is, as we know, characterized by its source, aim, and object. The relation to the object determines the developmental process. Mature, adult sexuality is an achievement, a result of libido's binding quality. Failure in this process can be seen in certain borderline conditions, where the difficulties in representing and relating to a whole object lead to display of partial self–object relations with acting out of relational needs, prominence of polymorph perverse sexual drives or perversions with fixation on part-aspects as the dominant means for satisfaction.

Consider what Freud writes in *Three Essays*: "one of our most surprising findings [was] that this early efflorescence of infantile sexuality (between the ages of two and five) already give rise to the choice of objects, with all the wealth of mental activities which such a process involves" (1905d, p. 158).

Shortly afterwards Freud comments on the two-phase onset of sexual development (childhood and adolescence, interrupted by a period of latency), saying that this biphasic development "appears to be one of the necessary conditions of the aptitude of men for developing a higher civilization, but also for their tendency to neurosis" (p. 158).

This civilizing capability is characterized by an increasing importance being given to the object relative to the aim of the drive or the release of tension.

The implication that the object is in a way an aspect of the drive and that the relation to and representation of the object is brought about by the work instigated by the drive has caused controversies. It was felt that an object only constituted by the drive itself represented an insufficient understanding of development, which then led to attempts at defining the role and influence of the relationship to the *external* object in development. Object seeking was thus separated from the influence of the drives. These longstanding differentiated relations to external objects and their mutual influence are, however, it could be argued, internalized and moulded by the drives and in that process come to constitute the building blocks of personality structure—or, as Freud's said in 1923: "the character of the ego is the precipitate of abandoned object cathexes and (that it) contains the history those object choices" (Freud, 1923b).

There are several problems involved here:

Do we need a separate theory of a "primary need for relationships"? Are the attempts to desexualize these primary relationship needs based on an insufficient understanding of sexuality and, for that reason, a restricted reading of the *Three Essays*? What is the relation between this need for a relationship with an object and the sexual aspects of relationships? Are these different or separate developmental paths to maturity (Emde, 1991)? And, finally, how do we work when relations are not symbolized or represented—that is, when there is a gap or insufficient grounds for interpretative work in the classical sense due to a lack of fantasies? And how do we understand the erotization of relationships that may follow? These are questions that are only partially answered within the developmentalist and attachment tradition, which in its pure cognitivistic approach does not consider personality to result from "object cathexes" and "object choices".

Seduction

In this context, Haynal's reflections on the mutual seduction in analysis are important: "what greater seduction is there than to offer to listen, attentively, four or five times a week, and thus become, on a regular basis, the centre of interest for the Other—who knows about failed seductions, and how these failures can become traumatic?" (Haynal, this chapter)

Seduction is, of course, understood not as the "gross seduction" of incest, but as the establishment of a libidinal bond, a complicated affective phenomenon communicated predominantly via emotional, non-verbal channels, taking place "in the triangle of sexuality, fantasy, and emotional experience".

Libido is generally responsible for the bonding between persons; it is behind the creation of the bond between mother and child and is present in all relationships, including the psychoanalytic. In Haynal's opinion this "fine libidinal force" needs rehabilitation in psychoanalysis—a claim that again challenges attachment theorists.

He argues that many analysts' primary occupation with the analysis of defences has shifted attention from understanding the sexual material or autoerotism that pervades the psychoanalytic situation and life in general. This brings the danger of an "obsessionalization" and intellectualization that may lead to a "drying out of the dynamics of the material".

This is in line with the claim, especially by French psychoanalysts, that sexuality is disappearing from psychoanalytic discourse and the observation that sexuality is mentioned less and less in psychoanalytic case reports (Green, 1995).

There is obviously an implied critique of ego psychology here, and perhaps also of the attachment-developmentalist approach, with its stress on mentalization and the cognitive aspect of development and psychoanalytic work. There seems, however, to be a development, among others, with theories on affective mentalization and attempts to place sexuality into an attachment context (Fonagy, Gergely, Jurist, & Target, 2002).

Fantasy

In his section on fantasy, Haynal, following Stoller (1979b), puts forward the idea that hostility is the driving force in desire and excitement in an attempt to undo childhood traumas and frustrations, and he asks whether the element of "bonification" in sexuality may have a similar function in restoring psychic balance as dream work may have when it succeeds in overcoming traumatic elements activated by daily events.

Here sexuality is understood not only as the motivating and organizing force that structures personality and pathology, but also as an ongoing activity doing psychic reparative work. The aim of sexuality is not just the release of tension; it is expressed, when repressed and hindered, in symptoms and character traits, or in perversions, as the direct expression of raw impulses.

In the clinic one can see here a distinction in relation to certain Kleinian approaches where the aggressive or hostile expressions in the dyad are focused and where an element of enduring, long-standing mental pain is often understood as being necessary for a successful analysis. This again is highly dependent on the analyst's ability to contain and do the work of reverie—an approach seemingly quite different from the playful approach that seems to pervade André Haynal's clinical attitude and work.

This brings to the front Eros and Thanatos, or the death drive—and the question of where to place desire, sexuality, and the seeking of ecstasy: what role do the death drive and aggressive drives play in sexuality? It is obvious that sexual practice is not necessarily a playful libidinal activity; it may be pervaded by aggression and attempts at overcoming infantile losses and traumas by creating scenarios that simultaneously fulfil intimate needs and express negative feelings towards the object. Haynal says that libido is responsible for bonding between persons, while the death drive (instinct) causes distance, repulsion, and hostility. While it is easy to agree with the importance of libidinal forces for creating bonds between people, one could here suspect a reification of the drives as separate forces in the mind operating out of any context of real frustration and gratification.

A central Freudian contribution is the understanding that sexuality, although a "product" of nature, is shaped and defined more by culture. Moreover, sex is a powerful organizer of experience, as Haynal also states. Bodily sensations and sensual pleasure define one's skin, and our boundaries and our relation to others are thus formed by the way sexuality shapes fantasies and the structure of the inner world.

Sexuality is, accordingly, both present as result of acculturation and formed in the same organizing experience. But, as far as formal research is concerned, could we then say that sexuality has an explanatory power? What is the role of motivation based on sexual drives as an explanation in a scientific argument? This should be an important question for the research community. Reading research reports, one gets the impression that even though sexuality may be seen as central, it is often relegated to metapsychological speculation and is given little place in the real scientific endeavour, except when explaining sexual perversions. While Freud saw his contribution in the *Three Essays* (1905d) as a dialogue with and an extension of the theories of the sexologists of the time and thus placed his work in a scientific context, it may seem that sexuality now has lost this footing in psychoanalytic science and research, while the scientific research on sexuality has again been left to the sexologists. The chapters in this book are, of course, a testimony to the contrary, but they may represent a minority voice within the psychoanalytic research community.

Gender theory

When mentioning gender theory, it may seem somewhat surprising that Haynal chooses to focus on rituals around childbirth and its significance for men. The difficulties of paternity reveal themselves in our culture in a possible increase in divorce and adultery by men in this period. Some non-Western cultures take care of these matters with certain rituals, again underlining the anthropological perspective and man's anchoring in culture.

Couvade refers to the custom that can be seen in certain "primitive" communities, where around the birth of a child the father takes to his bed for some time, keeps to a restricted diet, and performs rituals that mimic the labour of the woman giving birth.

Similar phenomena have been observed in Western cultures, but they are then medicalized and seen as an expression of somatized anxiety, pseudo-sibling rivalry, identification with the foetus, ambivalence about fatherhood, a statement of paternity, or parturition envy.

From an anthropological perspective it is, in this context, interesting to discuss the new developments in gender theory aimed at understanding the quite different appearance of sexuality and gender in Western cultures. For example, several studies have demonstrated striking differences in "gender behaviour" among fathers-to-be and new fathers even within Europe. For two generations now young men in the Nordic countries have participated from early on in "maternal" care, whereas England, for example, seems to lag one generation behind. Is this the influence of culture on gender behaviour, accidental different appearances of the same gender problem, or just a lack of kindergartens? Or are we seeing state-sponsored couvade rituals in the Nordic countries, an expression of social democratic libidinal force assimilating the rituals of couvades into modern culture?

Implication for research

Neglecting the sexual dimension may lead to an exclusively phenomenological understanding of the discourse of the analysand, Haynal claims.

In line with this, it is pertinent to ask whether observational empirical research into the psychoanalytic process or on psychoanalytic material may often, due to the method of research, lead to and solidify this intellectualization and "obsessionalization" that Haynal warns against—after all, we know researchers to be rather obsessional, and the methods used should be quite rigorous. If that is the case, what should be done? Will there be research strategies that can take complex motivational forces, and first and foremost sexuality, into account?

Freud argued for a combination of psychoanalytic investigation and observational studies and was well aware of the weaknesses of each method. Would that be a way forward, and how should such collaborative effort be accomplished?

There is now a demand for evidence-based medicine, and the "gold standard" is set by the randomized controlled design or the experiment that may be replicated. While it is obviously necessary to demonstrate the efficacy of psychoanalysis by the rigour of quantitative designs (the Stockholm study on outcome of psychoanalysis is an example of this, although it does not come up to "gold standard"—Sandell, Blomberg, Lazar, Carlsson, Broberg, & Schubert, 2000), empirical research has been criticized for not capturing the essence of psychoanalytic material. This critique is, in my opinion, misplaced, as it does not take into account the need for several research approaches within psychoanalysis. The qualitative approach, widely used in other disciplines and increasingly acknowledged in psychoanalysis, has the advantage of being able to follow the "fine threads" of intimate dialogues while at the same time representing scientific rigour, although not at the same level as numbers and data in quantitative empirical research. May I suggest this as a research approach more in the spirit of Haynal's perspective on psychoanalysis? Qualitative research takes complexity into account; it produces results not at the level of variations and combinations of data, but at the level of phenomena seen in context; it does not produce quantifiable results but is concerned with processes and tendencies that may be verified by the practising psychoanalyst (Varvin, 2003).

Cases

Haynal ends with some very interesting case vignettes that underscore the pervasiveness of infant sexuality or autoerotism in the manifestations of character and behaviour: the young man with his need for passive satisfaction, and the Don Juan in constant fear of being alone. This last is understood as a claim for a maternal presence as opposed to the unavailability of certain sexual objects. But could it not be interpreted as a use of sexuality to satisfy his primary need for a relationship? Again this poses the question of whether it is bonding or relational needs or sexuality that comes first.

Conclusion

André Haynal states that sexuality is the link to the innermost personality, to the real self; he claims, further, that "the lack of this perspective" may be the reason in many places for the diminishing interest in psychoanalysis. This is certainly true in a general sense. But this real self, is it only the self that was constituted in the sensuous relation to the other, beyond the self that has a primary need for a relation? Or is the last fiction an unnecessary construct that has brought psychoanalysis away from its grounding in infant sexuality? Is the development in our research and theories the last 100 years only a detour?

Psychoanalysis has revolutionized the view of humans as rooted in both nature and culture. Modern science, neuroscience, genetics, have taught us that nature is more rooted in culture than we had believed. Gender research has demonstrated that sexuality and gender are social constructions that, although rooted in nature, are formed by the social and cultural context. Research in psychoanalysis is necessary and formal empirical outcome research is mandatory now more than ever. We need, however, to preserve psychoanalysis as a science of man's sexual nature, how the drives form and are formed by relationships and historical/social context. And some research approaches are more "sexy" than others.

"Plus ça change, plus c'est la même chose"?

Haynal's chapter certainly reminds us of the fundamentals in psychoanalysis, clinically, theoretically, and, it is to be hoped, also for research.

3

Psychodynamic and biographical roots of a transvestite development: clinical and extra-clinical findings from a psychoanalysis

Marianne Leuzinger-Bohleber

Clinical, conceptual, and empirical research in psychoanalysis

As André Haynal has described in his chapter, social factors have changed in the century since Freud's *Three Essays on the Theory of Sexuality* (1905d), influencing—among other things—our view on what could be considered "normal" and what as "deviant" sexual behaviour.

Transvestite patients, like "Mr M", about whom I speak in this chapter, react seismographically to individual and social developments and changes in the realm of sexuality, attachment, and gender; hence I focus on this issue first. But as my professional competence is mainly in the field of *research* in psychoanalysis and not in social psychology, cultural studies, or anthropology, I concentrate on the illustration of the current position in the Research Subcommittee for Conceptual Research: that the three branches of clinical, conceptual, and empirical research in psychoanalysis can supplement each other in a productive way.

Therefore, first I present one aspect of clinical research that focuses on the psychodynamic and biographical roots of a transvestite development based on clinical findings of a five-year high-frequency psychoanalysis and a recent follow-up 24 years after termination of treatment. In a second part I summarize some of the conceptual reconsiderations concerning the psychodynamics, the biographical roots, and the psychic function of this sexual deviation and report on an interdisciplinary, empirically based conceptual research on memory, trying to illustrate that those interdisciplinary research findings may be helpful to conceptualize and to understand clinical material more precisely and deeply.

As Haynal discusses in his historical chapter, Freud did not differentiate between sex and gender. Money, Hampson, and Hampson (1955a, 1955b, 1956) developed this differentiation in their important studies on hermaphroditism. The important step in the gender differentiation can be seen in that the child develops a concordance between his/her—biological—sex and the sex of assignment and rearing: the child's gender. The gender differentiation is stabilized at around 18 months and finally at the age of around 4½. Stoller (1968) created the term "core-gender identity".

Because of space constraints, I am unable to summarize here the results of an extra-clinical, empirical study of the diary of this patient in which he had recorded each of his 624 analytic sessions. I have reported in other papers (Leuzinger-Bohleber, 1987, 1989; Leuzinger-Bohleber & Kächele, 1988) that a theory-guided, computer-supported content analysis of the changes in the manifest dream content, as well as the way the analysand was dealing with his dreams in the first 100 compared with the last 100 psychoanalytic sessions, showed a progressive and successful improvement of cognitive-affective problem-solving with unconscious material—the dreams. (Also because of limitations of space, authors and researchers dealing with related issues are cited in the References and Bibliography, but without details about their work.)

Psychoanalysis with a transvestite patient: one aspect of clinical psychoanalytical research

During recent decades the psychoanalytic community has become increasingly aware of the necessity for psychoanalysis to be more open to an interdisciplinary dialogue with other scientific disciplines as well as to empirical extraclinical research, without, on the other hand, renouncing the idiosyncrasy of psychoanalytic insight or its specific research field and methodology. Therefore, extra-clinical empirical research is indispensable for the development of psychoanalysis as a scientific discipline and for the dialogue with the non-psychoanalytic scientific world. The above-mentioned empirical study of the diary of the analysis of Mr M was part of an extra-clinical approach to the psychoanalytic process and its outcome (empirical single case studies as contributions to psychoanalytic outcome research—see, e.g., Cooper, 1991; Cooper, Kernberg, & Person, 1989; Holt, 1992; Leuzinger-Bohleber, Dreher, & Canestri, 2003; Leuzinger-Bohleber, Schneider, & Pfeifer, 1992; Modell, 1984; Sandler & Dreher, 1991; Thomä & Kächele, 1985; Wallerstein, 1988).

Nevertheless, the following insights into the unconscious determinants of the transvestite state of mind of Mr M and his dominant modality of sexual satisfaction could not have been discovered by any research method other than the clinical psychoanalytical one. I have summarized the psychoanalytic insights into the unconscious psychodynamic motives that determined the perversion of this patient as we have come to understand it in the intensive and to me impressive five-year psychoanalysis in a case study—a "novel", the traditional form of communication (of knowledge) within the psychoanalytic community. (We find quite a number of psychoanalytic case reports with transvestite or transsexual patients—e.g. by Busch de Ahumada, 2003, Calogeras, 1987; Coltart, 1985; Désirat, 1985; Fenichel, 1930; Francesconi, 1984; Glasser, 1979; Grand, 1997; Greenson, 1966; Herold, 2004; Kirkpatrick & Friedmann, 1976; Küchenhoff, 1988; Leuzinger-Bohleber, 1984; Lewis, 1963; Lothstein, 1977, 1983; Lothstein & Levine, 1981; Luca, 2002; Meyenburg, 1992; Oppenheimer, 1989, 1991; Quinodoz, 1999; Schwöbel, 1960b; Socarides, 1970a; Springer, 1981; Stein, 1995; Thomä, 1957; Volkan, 1973).

Within the scope of this chapter I cannot cover this topic completely, but I would like to try to give a brief impression of some of the clinical findings concerning the unconscious fantasies connected to the transvestite state of mind. I agree with Mervin Glasser (1979), Ofra Eshel (2005), Ruth Stein (2005), and others that transvestism, like all perversions, cannot be regarded as a psychopathological symptom but has to be seen as a distinguishable diagnostic state with a very complex structure and its own characteristics.

Mr M

Mr M, a 24-year-old student, came looking for psychotherapeutic help mainly because of his transvestism: he could only satisfy himself sexually while wearing women's clothes, especially stockings, slips, and bra, pressing his penis between his thighs and rubbing it through women's nylon stockings. In addition, he had the compulsion to steal women's underwear in shopping centres or grasp under the skirts of women in public places, actions that had often brought him into dangerous and shameful social situations. He also suffered from serious psychosomatic symptoms, such as stomach complaints, eczemas, and sleeping disturbances. He was severely socially isolated and spent most of his time indulging in transvestite fantasies and actions. He was not able to study or to work at the time of the interviews.

Mr M was a very tall young man with broad shoulders, curly hair that looked a bit like Struwwelpeter's, and big blue eyes in a childlike face. The way he moved his body did not remind me of femininity but, rather, of a narcissistic cathexis of his own body. Following him up the stairs to my office, I had the fantasy that he was smoothly sliding or even flying, not really touching the stairs.

After having sat down—in *my* chair—for the initial interview, he said: "I am a narcissistic exhibitionistic transvestite." Then he handed me a 30-page manuscript: "Please study this. It is my biography. Writing it, I came to the conclusion that I need a psychoanalysis." It was not only this behaviour that looked very unusual to me. I also registered a very unusual countertransference fantasy of mine: I immediately experienced a strong aversive bodily reaction, connected to the thought: "Well, my dear: transvestism is a perversion after all: I will refer you to classic behavioural treatment!" At that time a student of mine had just studied the quite sadistic techniques of treating perverse patients with electroshock therapy, and so on, practised by some traditional behavioural therapists. Therefore, I was quite shocked by my sadistic countertransference fantasies and tried to understand their unusual intensity. I finally supposed that my aversive reactions on his enactment might be connected to his need to radically deny my existence as a separate person, an incontrollable

> object on whom he could depend: he was even able to formulate his diagnosis and the indication for psychoanalysis without any help from a professional! He also seemed to project unbearable feelings of impotence and despair and to dispose of them in me like a violent attempt to find—via projective identifications—a way to open a door to the psychic space of a closed-up, rejecting ego (Feldman, 1999, p. 1001).
>
> In later sequences of the interview I again noticed a strange bodily reaction: I suddenly felt sort of melted with Mr M—the boundaries between us seemed to blur. This was one reason for me to agree with his self-diagnosis: in my view, he suffered from a narcissistic personality disorder combined with perverse and psychosomatic symptoms, disturbances that could only be treated with long-term, intensive psychoanalysis. I expected the treatment to become rather difficult but possibly to turn out successful, because the patient seemed to be creative and gifted for psychoanalytic work.

I will concentrate on one aspect of the clinical research findings, the understanding of some aspects of the unconscious fantasies connected with transvestism, to summarize of some of the characteristics of *clinical psychoanalytic research, its idiosyncratic chances as well as its limits and even dangers.*

Transvestism: the unconscious fantasy to be an omnipotent man–woman

Transvestism, the unconscious fantasy to be an omnipotent man–woman, constitutes a narcissistic defence against the unbearable feeling of dependency on the (depressed) primary object.

As early as 1979, Glasser wrote that the mothers of perverts relate to their children narcissistically, as extensions of themselves, and so fail to recognize the child's own emotional needs, wishes, and cognitions. His transvestite analysand felt "enveloped" by women's clothes, with the implication that he would be annihilated. One of the core complexes was the fusion with the object—originally the idealized mother. Later Glasser (1992) spoke of a "colonizing pre-oedipal mother". The perverse and narcissistic kind of defence of the patient might be seen as an attempt to avoid further (traumatic) dependency on an object as well as an indicator for primary identifications with a narcissistic mother. Luca (2002) described the perverse manifestations in a therapy with a perverse patient with transvestite symptoms emerging as an inability to experience any affect. Another similarity between her clinical observations and mine is the immediate intensity of transference, although the manifestations of transference seemed to be quite different (see also Coltart, 1985). In Luca's therapy a seductive and erotized transference developed at once. Another analogy in the course of both treatments was that her patient as well as Mr M fell into a severe depression after the narcissistic and perverse defence was analysed in the transference (Luca, 2002, 657ff).

The unconscious enactments during the initial interview dominated in many sessions during the first year of treatment. Mr M's need to control the sessions—and me—characterized the first months: he began, shaped, and ended the sessions himself. For nearly a whole year he did not seem to be able to perceive me as an independent or even an interpreting object. Therefore, I was mostly silent or trying to take up some aspects in his thoughts, repeating them or—in some exceptions—formulating them in a slightly different way. Mr M always created interpretations by himself. I often had to think of the myth of Narcissus rejecting the passion of the Nymph Echo and instead falling passionately and deadly in love with himself, being fixed to staring at his face in the mirroring water. If ever—in analogy—in our analytic sessions I did not succeed in behaving as a perfect mirror or an "echo" for himself (as a self-object, see Kohut, 1971)—he reacted with much irritation—for example, as he expressed it once, "with a flight into women's clothes after the session". Of course, this enactment was not always easy to bear: I often registered severely aggressive countertransference feelings—for example, that a wax puppet could have sat behind the couch with a tape-recorded "Hmm . . ." instead of me. In other sequences of the sessions—again analogously to the initial interview—the inner boundaries between us seemed to blur. Sometimes I observed that I even took up psychosomatic symptoms, such as stomach-aches, from Mr M—at that time an uneasy and even scary experience for me. At the same time Mr M experienced himself consciously as the "best analysand" and me " as the best analyst of the world": an image of a narcissistic wholeness and unity, a fantasized paradise. Finally we understood a first meaning of the transvestite state of mind: wearing women's clothes symbolized a state of narcissistic omnipotence: to be simultaneously both man and woman (or a male analysand melted with a female analyst), a state of narcissistic self-nurturing, a narcissistic "envelope" (Gerzi, 2005) not dependent on anybody!

This narcissistic defence was obviously needed because of an extreme feeling of fragility and vulnerability. In the analytic sessions as well as in reality we were able to observe the extreme fear of being humiliated or exposed to situations of shame and blame. ("His fear of humiliation was also a central factor in his avoidance of getting in touch with any affect"—Luca, 2002, p. 657.) Shame was also the dominant affect in his initial dream (which he told me about in the tenth session):

"I am walking on a street between two red houses and carry a blanket with me. In one of the houses lives Rahel, my second girlfriend. I am entering the house of Rahel's mother and discover a crooked bed. It is standing on a hay barn. Suddenly I am lying on this bed, and Rahel's mother bows down to me. People are coming and laughing—yes, they laughed at Mrs X because she had sexual intercourse with me. I feel very embarrassed, and we both are hiding under the blanket. I then argue and defend myself: this is not true at all. I am getting up but don't wear any clothes. I am leaving, I put women's clothes on, and then I am suddenly on the deck of an ornate Mississippi steamer. Many people are dancing there. I have to demonstrate 'what I can do'. I am dancing, and then I am flying away. . . . "

The associations lead to different situations of shame in real life: such as Rahel's mother blaming him because he had not been able to construct a straight part in the planting area of the garden ("*schiefes Gartenbeet*", which means literally: a crooked garden bed). He also associated his fear to be exposed to shameful situations on the couch. Mr M often had dreams of flying, rescuing him—as in the initial dream—from such shameful or dangerous situations.

In the following weeks he also remembered some core scenes of his early childhood, when his mother had humiliated her husband in front of the children—probably "screen memories" of traumatic experiences of denigration and devaluation of himself by his mother.

The devaluation of the fathers by the mothers of these patients is described in other case reports on transvestite patients (e.g. Busch de Ahumada, 2003; Calogeras, 1987; Coltart, 1985; Grand, 1997; Luca, 2002), and Heinemann (1998) observed a cultural analogy in her ethnopsychoanalytic study in which she discovered frequent and culturally accepted transvestite developments in boys ["*fakafefine*"] in Tonga, Polynesia, a culture in which women seem to have more narcissistic and social acceptance than men. Thus, separation from the mothers is not attractive either for sons or for the mothers themselves, and transvestites remain living with their mothers, are involved in female activities, and are socially highly accepted and appreciated.

Later in analysis we found out that Mr M's mother had suffered from severe depressions during the first years of his life—a post-partum depression following a difficult birth. He was her second son. When he asked her, she told him that she could not cope with her disappointment that he was not the expected girl, but another boy. In the second year of M's life she gave birth to a third son, who died shortly after birth (because of an undiscovered genetic problem in the mother's family). Obviously the mother felt guilty for having caused this death and again fell into a severe depression. She had to be hospitalized for several months. The patient was brought to his grandparents and lived there for more than half a year.

Thus, the clinical research during the five years of analytic work revealed the severe early traumatizations that probably led Mr M to the above-mentioned narcissistic defence of the unbearable experience of dependency on a primary (depressed) object who, due to her severe depression, probably had not been capable of containing the early impulses and fantasies of her baby or empathizing in a "good-enough" way with his needs and inner states. The early object relation with his depressed mother thus did not enable Mr M to integrate the archaic psychic world into stable self- and object representations. His recurrent dreams during the first year of analysis hinted at this inner archaic mental world: he often woke up in panic because he was persecuted and bitten by horses or sharks or swallowed by elephants.

As Freud explained in his later theories of perversion and, after him, many theorists had elaborated: the perversion serves as a defence not only against severe castration anxieties but also against a regression into a psychotic state of the mind. Morgenthaler (1974) considered the perversion as a kind of a "*Plombe*" [filling (for tooth)] that ameliorated the unbearable feelings of narcissistic vulnerability and severe depression and thus prevented a psychotic fragmentation of the self. (According to Morgenthaler, this vulnerability has to be treated in analysis before working on the different meanings of the perversion; this is one reason why too early interpretations of libidinal and aggressive impulses in treatment often lead to a disruption of the treatment.)

Therefore, the first observable change after about 10 months of analysis was a decrease in Mr M's enormous vulnerability. He once expressed in the session that he now felt "more complete", "round", "a whole person", and he suffered less from fears of being blamed or exposed to shameful situations. This was also observable in the sessions: he could now endure that he was not able to control me all the time and that I could even say something unexpected to him. Parallel to this development, he experienced for the first time direct feelings of dependency on me. Before the first summer break he had a panic dream in which *his mother and I were hanging up wet clothes together. I told him that we could not continue with analysis because he had failed. The couch was lying in front of him, cut into three pieces.* Trying to understand this dream and his separation anxieties, we discovered another meaning of his transvestite state, which consider in the following section.

Transvestism as transitional object trying to cope with separation and individuation: disidentifying from the mother

Stoller (1968) and others discussed that—in contrast to Freud's concepts of the development of male or female identity—men have a more difficult development than women because they have to "disidentify" from their female primary object. Stoller talks of proto-femininity—a concept criticized by many—as one reason why men suffer more often from cross-gender identity problems than do women. Transsexuality occurs four times as frequently in men than in women. Transvestites (heterosexuals with fetishistic preferences for clothes of the other gender) is only found with men. Also, effeminate homosexuals are more often men (see Person & Ovesey, 1993, p. 518).

> A new memory occurred during these months: the transvestite symptoms had developed for the first time during a situation of separation in the fifth year of the patient's life.

Calogeras (1987) analysed a patient whose transvestite symptoms had also developed after being shut in a dark cellar between his third or fourth year of life. Grand (1997) published an analysis with a transvestite patient after a mother–son incest. The patient had slept for several years in the bed of his mother, who suffered from a severe depression after the death of her husband when the patient was 2 years old. Moguillansky's transvestite patient also had a depressed and alcoholic mother. He used masturbation in women's clothes as an anxiolytic or antidepressant. He was mute at home and was treated for this elective mutism for a short time at 6 years of age. He was in treatment again at the age of 17 due to his shyness and night fears. Francesconi (1984) treated a transvestite patient who tried to deny the separateness from his mother in the transvestite act. This act also served the fantasy that the primary object is under total control by the self. Like Mr M, her patient had an excessive relationship to a transitional object until adulthood. Meyer (1996) reported on a two-year psychotherapy with a transvestite patient (out of a sample of 500 patients with sexual disorders); according to his wide experiences, transvestites can integrate ambivalence between a part of themselves in connection with reality and another part with a psychotic denial of reality, while transsexuals cannot.

> When his parents went out at night, they locked M into their bedroom. There he discovered the underwear of his mother, put it on, and felt comfortable and consoled. Thus, his transvestite symptom had a similar function to a transitional object: it symbolized the closeness and the presence of the maternal primary object and thus helped in a creative act of imagination to deny separateness.

> Due to the just mentioned traumatizations, this denial of separateness had an archaic quality and was connected with extreme feelings of hatred and destructive aggression towards the primary object. In his transvestite behaviour he also enacted revenge on his primary object, as well as on women in general: he could control them by putting on their clothes—and he no longer needed women for his sexual satisfaction.
>
> In analysis, one of the most delicate sequences occurred in the second year while the separation conflicts connected with these extreme destructive fantasies seemed to be intensively activated in the transference. Mr M shocked me one day by telling me that he had fixed a date for a "sex-change operation". I was shocked not only by this fact and the extreme destructiveness against analysis by Mr M trying to destroy our treatment by this operation but also by my own countertransference reactions: I immediately observed strange and cold fantasies: "Well, if you want to do this operation, do whatever you want—but please after our treatment, I don't want to have anything to do with this. . . ." In my supervision we understood these fantasies as an indicator for the ongoing projective identifications in the transference as well as for the coldness and the lack of basic empathy by the depressed primary object. This insight helped me to regain my analytic attitude and to deal professionally with the delicate situation in analysis. Mr M then decided to defer his decision for a possible sex operation until the end of psychoanalysis.
>
> In the follow-up 24 years after termination, Mr M spontaneously recalled this delicate situation and told me how important it had been for him that he did not feel put under pressure from me. He told me that he has lived in a satisfactory marriage for 20 years now and has two adolescent children, a girl and a boy.

A stable marriage seems to be one indicator that the aim of marrying a woman was not primarily to stabilize the man's own fragile gender identity. As Calogeras (1987) and others report, if the later is the case, the marriage usually breaks down after a few months or years. Coltart (1985), in her extensive case report, discussed the enormous marital difficulties of a transvestite patient and his wife in the context of the shared wish to have a child. Although the couple—due to the analysis of the patient—

finally were able to have two children, the patient left his family afterwards. His problems with his identity as a father as well as a potent sexual partner did not allow him to live a "regular" family life.

> Mr M had a first serious crisis when his boy, the second child, was born, and he feared that he could not be an adequate father to him. He managed to overcome this crisis without professional help. The other serious crisis occurred during the adolescence of his son while one of his closest friends, a colleague at work, left his family, telling them that he was homosexual.
>
> "You know, I always realized that my transvestite wishes and desires have not disappeared completely, although I do live a normal sex life with my wife. I know it is still there somewhere in my soul. I often feel quite lonely with this part of mine—my wife does not want to hear anything about it. I have never have talked to anyone about it since my analysis. You have been the only person whom I took with me into this secret part of my soul. During my crisis, five years ago, I decided to try to get into contact with this side of mine again on my own. During my sabbatical I spent half a year in X [a town in Germany where I used to live after the termination of the analysis with Mr M] in a psychiatric hospital. I was in charge of a sensitivity group of transsexuals. It was a central experience for me, seeing that maybe for some of these patients the sex operation had been a solution. For myself, I realized that these persons don't live an easier life than I do—I think their lives must be even more complicated, because they are always living 'in-between': they are neither women nor men. Their fantasy to be able to change sex and gender has turned out to be an illusion. I felt so grateful that I had the possibility to discover and anticipate this problem in analysis. Thus, I think that each transsexual or transvestite patient should go into analysis before the definite decision to have an operation. Since these weeks in X, I am better able to live with my transvestite fantasies, and always ask myself what meanings my longings might have when they appear in a certain situation in my everyday life. . . ."

Quinodoz (1999) published an impressive case report with a transsexual patient who had undergone a sex operation and was living as a woman afterwards. She discusses her clinical observation that the patient used sexualization as a defence against a narcissistic wound and vulnerability. I cannot go deeper here into historical and current discussions on transsexuality (see, e.g., Braun-Scharm & Loeben-Sprengel, 1988; Burzig, 1982; Chiland, 1998; Herold, 2004; Hertrampf, 1999; Pfäfflin, 1993, 2003). I only want to mention that, according to Pfäfflin (1994), about one third of transsexual patients decide not to undergo a sex-change operation during and after psychotherapy.

> It turned out that Mr M wanted to contact me again because he was uncertain whether he should share his "transvestite secret" with his children, particularly with his son.
>
> He also expressed his mourning and sadness that his mother had not been able to accept his male sex and had thus disturbed a normal male gender development—one reason for his overstimulated aggressive feelings towards women.

Most such parents, particularly the mothers, seem unable to accept and enjoy the male sex of their transvestite sons (see, e.g., Calogeras, 1987; Luca, 2002).

> Mr M recalled another sequence of analysis during the second year of treatment, when he had discovered a photo of himself as a five-year-old child, dressed up as a girl. His mother had confessed to him that at that time she had often dressed him up as a girl because "you looked so cute as a girl. . . ."
>
> In my view, Mr M had thus suffered from Type II trauma, according to Terr (1991)—a chronic form of trauma that is due to a pathological object relation with the depressed and probably perverse mother who had probably mainly failed in her basic holding and containing functions for her baby boy. Another pathogenic factor was probably connected to the fact that his father was not able to function in a "good-enough way" as an attractive, secure, and compensating fatherly object and identification figure either during the early triangulation or during the oedipal phase or in adolescence.

Transvestism and castration anxiety

Mr M also suffered from Type I traumatizations (Terr, 1991). I can only mention one example here: during his fifth year of life M—while playing football with his elder brother—had a serious car accident with a contusion and complicated broken leg. In the third year of analysis he remembered that he had developed an encopresis during his long stay in the hospital, and a nurse had threatened him: "If you are lying and deny that the excrements in your bed are yours, your leg will never be cured." In many dreams and associations we discovered an unconscious truth that had probably developed during this developmental phase: "As a boy you can lose your penis! To wear women's clothes may have the meaning—look at me: I don't have a penis, therefore I am already castrated. . . ." (As in the initial dream, where his girlfriend's mother was bowing down to him, Mr M often dreamt of women with a penis, probably a manifestation of the unconscious fantasy of the phallic woman—see Chasseguet-Smirgel, 1980.)

After his traumatic experiences stimulating the oedipal castration anxieties as well as the early separation conflicts, the transvestite symptoms developed during the above mentioned situation of separation.

Because of space limitations I can only mention and not discuss some of the other unconscious meanings of the transvestite state of mind that we discovered in our clinical work.

- *The girl—a protection against maternal death wishes.* An unconscious fantasy system developed in the context of fantasies around the death of his second baby brother and the depression of the mother.
- *Transvestism as revenge towards the neglecting primary object—and thus women in general—as well as towards the missing fatherly identification figure.* The transvestite patient described by Francesconi (1984) seems to wear women's clothes because he had the illusion as a girl he would be loved by everybody. He was rejected by his mother and given to his grandparents shortly after his birth.
- *Transvestism: a narcissistic defence after renewed traumatizations during adolescence and seismographic reactions to modern gender conflicts.*

Interdisciplinary, empirically based conceptual research: transvestism and perversion

André Haynal has already summarized Freud's *Three Essays on the Theory of Sexuality* (1905d) and his conceptualization of sexual deviation as well as the development of theories on sexual deviation (as transvestism) in the psychoanalytic literature during the last 100 years in his contribution in this volume. Therefore, I can refer to his chapter and return, instead, to the relationship between clinical, conceptual, and empirical research as we have discussed it in detail elsewhere (see Leuzinger-Bohleber & Bürgin, 2003, Leuzinger-Bohleber, Fischmann, & Research Committee for Conceptual Research, in press).

Clinical research in psychoanalysis

I have just presented some aspects of the circular clinical research that is understood as a never-ending circular process that can be characterized by, on the one hand, the artful clinical attempt to meet the analysand in each session with an open mind, an attitude of "not knowing", and, on the other—as we discussed in the paper just mentioned (Leuzinger-Bohleber & Bürgin, 2003)—our clinical understanding always depends, of course, on the quality of the concepts behind it in our minds: the higher their quality, the better the perception of the complexity of our clinical material. What were the concepts of the psychodynamics and the unconscious biographical determinants of the transvestite state of my patient when I first published the case novel in 1984? At that time I understood the biographical background of the transvestite development mainly in the context of severe traumatizations during the oedipal phase on the one hand and during the phase of separation–individuation on the other. With this conceptualization I was in agreement with most psychoanalysts who had published papers on the psychodynamics and the biographical roots of transvestite patients.

To summarize briefly my original interpretations of the clinical findings:

1. The transvestite symptoms developed in Mr M's sixth year of life: After a traumatic accident and hospitalization he discovered,

having been locked into the bedroom of his parents, his mother's underwear, put it on, and felt comforted, sexually stimulated, and relieved from his painful feelings of being all alone and in a completely impotent, helpless situation. After this event he asked for nappies in games with other children and stole female underwear.

As the development of the symptoms illustrates: M failed to master the oedipal conflict in a "good-enough way":

The accident was a traumatic event for him and deepened his castration anxieties (he remembered the threat by the nurse: if you are lying, your leg will never be cured again). His mother's underwear (and later women's underwear in general) became a symbol for a protection of his threatened penis. His symptom also seemed to mean: "Look at me: I am already a woman: I don't have a penis. Therefore, I cannot be castrated any more!" Thus—symbolically—he actively castrated himself instead of enduring the risk of being (passively) castrated.

The symptom of compulsively grasping under the skirts of women in public places had a similar meaning: He wanted to protect the woman's vagina and to assert himself at the same time—there is no difference between her and myself (the woman had to wear panties): Men and women are alike!

In this context it is important to mention that his father was not available for M "in a good-enough way" as an oedipal identification figure during his early childhood . Some indicators for this hypothesis: the father was often devalued and humiliated by his wife, he had not been accepted by the Swiss Army, and he worked below his professional qualification.

2. The nine weeks of hospitalization after the accident reactivated the early separation traumata: In his second year of life his baby brother died shortly after birth. The mother felt guilty and narcissistically injured and had to be hospitalized in a psychiatric clinic. M was brought to his grandparents. In many dreams we discovered the "unconscious truth" that his baby brother had died because of his jealousy and because of his mother's anger and disappointment that he was a boy and not the desired girl. In this context wearing women's clothes meant: "Being a girl, you

are loved and accepted by the mother—as a boy, you can lose your penis and your life."

The depression of the mother also made M's separation and individuation very difficult: she was probably not able to enjoy his growing up experiencing him as a separate and autonomous self. I was not able to summarize the impressive clinical findings here: in the third year of analysis Mr M seemed convinced that he had destroyed me during the summer holidays because—for the first time—he had enjoyed being separated from me, and he "did his own things". Many nightmares illustrated his archaic mental world in which the murderous oral and anal aggressive libidinal impulses dominated: snakes, sharks, elephants, lions, and rhinos were pursuing him, swallowing him or tearing him to pieces. He also suffered from extreme sadistic fantasies that had also been reactivated in the transference—e.g. in the context of his planned sex operation. He often dreamt that his penis was a knife that destroyed his love object or himself.

We also assumed that the transvestite symptom was connected to the fantasy that his depressed mother could not love him as a separate, "big boy": He had the fantasy that he could replace the dead baby brother and the fantasized baby girl for his mother by wearing girls' clothes (photographs of being dressed up as a girl). Thus, the transvestite state guaranteed the symbiotic closeness to his mother on the one hand, while, at the same time, by wearing his mother's clothes, he was able to comfort himself independently of her in the situation of separateness, thus proving that he did not need her any more: "Well, if you really want it: I am playing the girl for you, but what I am really thinking and feeling behind these clothes will never be transparent to you any more. . . ." In contrast to transsexual patients, M experienced ambivalence: he knew that he was a man even while feeling the longing to "be a woman".

In psychoanalysis it became clear that the father was mostly absent during the early period of life: he was also hardly fulfilling the role of the third in the early triangulation phase. He could thus not sufficiently support the separation from the maternal primary object. The father was a very creative person, who constructed organs in the basement—a fantastic world for both of

> his boys. But at the same time he was the devaluated object of the mother and thus not an attractive identification figure for M. Nevertheless we supposed that Mr M's talent for fantasizing and writing was connected to early unconscious identification with his creative father.

Although—two decades ago—I was quite sure about the role of this "double sequence of traumatizations" for the development of the transvestite symptoms, even at that time I was looking for a third possible source of transvestism.

I wrote that I was uncertain why Mr M had developed a narcissistic kind of defence—"the narcissistic envelope" according to Gerzi (2005)—as we had observed it during the first year of analysis. Which had been the unconscious determinants of the extreme psychic retreat (John Steiner, 1993) of my patient? How could his obvious fragility, vulnerability, and depression, connected to the archaic mental world of destructiveness and fragmentation, be understood? Was his psychic state more or less exclusively due to the above mentioned traumatic conflicts during the separation–individuation phase (according to Margaret Mahler), or had there been traumatic experiences in the early object relationships? At that time I only knew for certain that M had been born too early, that his birth had been quite dramatic, and that his mother suffered from a postpartum depression.

On the basis of the findings of a large number of clinical and empirical studies over the last 20 years, we can answer these questions much more precisely now—in other words, this broadened knowledge may be part of further *conceptual research on the psychodynamics and the development of a transvestite state of mind.*

Conceptual research integration: further clinical research in psychoanalysis

In this period many psychoanalytic clinical papers have been published focusing the early object relation between the infant and a depressed primary object (see, e.g., Cooper, Kernberg, & Person, 1989; Eshel, 2005; Fonagy & Target, 1997; Gerzi, 2005; Green, 1999; Kohon, 1999; Leuzinger-Bohleber, 2001; Stein, 2005; for other titles see starred entries listed in the References and Bibliography).

Conceptual research based on further extraclinical, empirical research

Daniel Stern related these clinical findings—for example, the concept of the "dead mother" by André Green—with the findings of empirical infant research on early interactions with a depressed primary object. He showed that these early infantile experiences do have a traumatic quality for the development of a stable core self of the infant (see, e.g., Stern, 1995). He defined four typical schemata "of being with a depressed mother" which have since been widely discussed:

1. the infant's experience of repeated "microdepression"
2. the infant's experience of being a reanimator
3. the experience of "mother as a background in seeking stimulation elsewhere"
4. the experience of an inauthentic mother and self

It goes beyond the scope of this chapter to discuss the relevance of these four schemata for a deeper understanding of the transvestite development of Mr M and other perverse patients. I only want to mention that I was able to reconstruct traces of all four different schemata in the enactment of Mr M in the course of his analysis: the identification with the depression of the primary object, his attempt to vitalize a "dead maternal object", his flight into autoerotic stimulation (particularly skin and body stimulation) by putting on women's clothes as a replacement for a stimulating and satisfying interaction with a primary (nondepressed) object (Type 3) and the development of a false, inauthentic self (for my hypotheses on the narcissistic transvestite personality and the deep identity conflicts of Mr M, see Leuzinger-Bohleber & Pfeifer, 1998, pp. 904ff.).

Interdisciplinary, empirically based conceptual research

Our attempt to integrate these empirical findings conceptually with clinical psychoanalytical knowledge as well as with findings of other disciplines in the field of memory research—for example, the so-called Embodied Cognitive Science—is, I think, less well known, and hence I will illustrate briefly (as one example of the so-called *interdisciplinary, empirically based conceptual research*) how this knowledge might contribute to a deeper understanding of some of the early biographical roots of the transvestite development or Mr M and other patients.

The conceptualization is based on an interdisciplinary dialogue that I have conducted with Rolf Pfeifer, Professor of Cognitive Science at the University of Zurich, for more than 20 years, above all on subjects such as memory, remembering, transference, and working-through in the analytic relationship (see Leuzinger-Bohleber & Pfeifer, 2002; Pfeifer & Leuzinger-Bohleber, 1986; among others). In some of our papers we have been concerned with the question just mentioned—namely, how early memories of a depressive primary object must be conceptualized from the point of view of a dialogue on memory between psychoanalysis and Embodied Cognitive Science. In one of these papers we take up a controversial discussion on the role of early "historical" experiences for memories and unconscious determinants of psychopathological symptoms. Some colleagues, such as Peter Fonagy and Mary Target (1997), deny that historical reality is central for the understanding of the early roots in the sufferings of our patients. They write in their summary: ". . . whether there is historical truth and historical reality is not our business as psychoanalysts and psychotherapists" (p. 216). In his keynote lecture at the Forty-fourth IPA Congress on Trauma in Rio de Janeiro Peter Fonagy (2005) elaborates and differentiates his position again:

> The frontal lobes appear to play a key role in monitoring the source of a memory image, including distinguishing true and false memories; prior expectations can create an unusually vivid set of ideas or images. The hyperactivation of the attachment system in individuals with trauma and the likely associated inhibition of mentalizing may compromise source monitoring. The focus by a therapist on recreating and reviving memories will inevitably introduce a further bias. This is a possibility rather than a demonstrated fact. However, the therapist must be aware that the cognitive monitoring functions normally available to individuals to prevent confusion between fantasy and memory may be specifically compromised by the therapeutic process itself. Nevertheless, I believe that reconstruction is essential to the therapeutic process itself because (1) it provides a means to bring the patient's mind into contact with what has previously found intolerable; (2) it provides a place where threat to the ego and therapeutic goal are reasonably balanced; (3) it generates

> a coherent self narrative assuming a historical continuity of self which may itself be of therapeutic value (Spence, 1982); (4) it can help in primary task of the recovery of mentalization. [p. 22 of unpublished manuscript]

In spite of this differentiation, for Fonagy the primary task of a psychoanalytic process is mentalization. To approach historical truth has only a subordinate meaning and remains risky. The argument developed above, taking into account findings from Embodied Cognitive Science, offers a different perspective on the task: that not only narrative but historical truth as well is essential for a psychoanalytic process. Fonagy and Target argue that many memory researchers have postulated in recent years that declarative (autobiographical) and procedural (implicit) memory must be distinguished from each other (see also summaries by Köhler, 1998, and by Mertens, 1998, among others). On a descriptive level this differentiation makes sense: in the declarative memory we store verbal, visual, and symbolic memories; in the procedural memory we store memories of physical processes that cannot become conscious in later periods of time. Our 20-year-old daughter remembers, for instance, being held by her father when learning to ski at the age of 3. However, it is almost impossible for her as an adolescent to remember the exact motor skills she learned then and that she still (unconsciously) performs. Declarative memory—which the neuroscientist Gerhard Roth (2001) calls the predominantly responsible region of the hippocampus—does not develop until the third or fourth year of life, and for Fonagy and Target this represents the argument why memories cannot cover experiences of the first three years. Rolf Pfeifer and I have questioned this conclusion. We have argued that the *differentiation between declarative and procedural memory refers to the descriptive level of memory performance and not to processes in the brain that enable remembering.* Even if the region of the hippocampus is not fully developed until the third or fourth year of life, experiences are nevertheless stored in the brain structures before then, even in their entirety and not just in a single, specific brain region. (The so-called "localization thesis" is seen as outdated today, although certain regions of the brain are, of course, connected to certain psychic processes in a particularly intensive way—see, e.g., Damasio, 1994; Edelman, 1987, 1992; Kaplan-Solms & Solms, 2000; Roth, 2001.) Our arguments are based on research in Embodied Cognitive Science. Dowling (1989) has discussed a similar position, taking up Piaget's studies on sensorimotor organization: "Sensory motor mentation, like every early organization, continues as a non-dominant mode throughout life" (p. 95). The concept of "embodiment" postulates—in contrast to his view—that early, preverbal experiences do play a central role during the whole of life. The storehouse metaphor is still often found in the literature of academic psychology, as we have discussed elsewhere (see Leuzinger-Bohleber & Pfeifer, 2002, pp. 7–9). Moreover, in some papers the representation model of psychoanalysis is understood according to the idea that early experiences are engraved on the memory (see also Freud's "*Wunderblock*" or Aristotle's' metaphor of the memory as a wax tablet).

According to Embodied Cognitive Science, memory and remembering should no longer be conceived as stored structures in the sense of a "storehouse model" (computer metaphor) but, rather, as knowledge that is stored in what is called declarative memory after the third year of life and that can be retrieved in a new, structurally analogous situation, like pressing a button on a computer and so transferring knowledge from long-term to short-term memory. This notion of memory has proven to be false: human memory functions analogously not to a computer but to a biological self-regulating system that constantly adapts to new and changing environments! According to biological memory research, remembering has now to be understood as a function of the whole organism: as a complex, dynamic recategorizing and interactive process that is always *"embodied"*—in other words, is based on sensorimotor experiences—and that becomes manifest in the behaviour of the organism, not just in the brain or in a specific region in the brain. These memory concepts have been experimentally tested in the field of Embodied Cognitive Science by robotics, a field of experimental and empirical research that is not very widely known (see, e.g., Pfeifer & Scheier, 1999); the research teams of Gerald D. Edelman and Antonio Damasio also apply this experimental method in order to test their models of memory.

This means that memory is not an abstract cognitive function; it is always based on actual sensorimotor stimulations that receive and process visual, haptic, auditory, and proprioceptive stimuli and, as in earlier situations, actively make up and "produce" out of them analogies between the current and this earlier situation—memories. Thus, "embodied" remembering is not simply "non-verbal" or "descriptively unconscious" but highly constructive, dynamic, and historically determined.

To give an example: in the initial interview with Mr M, I unconsciously received information from many different channels—visual (e.g. the narcissistic body movements of Mr M, his male body, child-like face, big blue eyes, etc.), haptic (the way, Mr M shook my hands or handed his manuscript to me, my own bodily receptions sitting in the patient's chair instead of in my own, etc.), auditory (I noticed that Mr M proposed his own diagnosis and indication, but also how nonverbally he seemed to deny that I was even listening to him: he preached in some way to an unknown audience and did not try to communicate with me as an idiosyncratic individual), and so on. Unconsciously I coordinated the information from all these different sensory channels and "constructed" a strong negative bodily reaction, which was then—also unconsciously—associated with my cold and unempathetic thought: "Well, my dear: transvestism is a perversion, after all: I will refer you to classic behavioural treatment!" My thesis is that these were countertransferential reactions to the unconscious transference signals that Mr M enacted in his sensorimotor co-ordination in the interaction with me (sending the above mentioned signals via the different channels, which I perceived unconsciously). In the "here-and-now" of the initial interview (objectively seen in a dependent position with an "Important Other") unconscious memories engraved in his body were activated and determined his enactment. To describe it verbally: as we know from traumatized patients, Mr M tried to convert the traumatic experience from a passively suffered one into an actively produced one. As his depressed primary object, he denied, in a cold, unempathetic manner, my existence as an independent personality, putting me (in place of himself) into an absolutely helpless, useless position, analogous to the position of a helpless baby that is not accepted the way it is, with his sex, his needs, and his wish to interact with a competent, warm, secure, and helpful person. To formulate it metaphorically: by way of the mechanism of projective identification he then experienced me, as illustrated by my countertransference reactions, analogously to his primary object, which—due to postpartum depression—had not been able to be sensitive enough towards the needs and impulses of the baby but basically rejected and neglected it.

In psychoanalysis we would describe these processes as introjective and projective identifications. The concept of "embodiment" seems to be able to add a dimension of explanation to our psychoanalytic concepts. Verbal and bodily countertransference reactions are not mysterious in any sense: they could principally be observed by detailed mini-analyses of the stimuli in the different channels of Mr M which were then perceived by me and—in the sense of sensorimotor coordination—led to the "construction" of extreme aversive bodily reactions and cold and rejecting countertransference fantasies. (I think, for example, of the micro-analyses of the exchange of facial signals, which the research team of Rainer Krause in Saarbrücken or Eva Bänninger-Huber in Innsbruck have been conducting for years.)

Thus, according to the memory concepts of Embodied Cognitive Science, early object relations experiences influence the neural network and are engraved in the "hardware" of the body. Afterwards they will determine perceptions and affects in new interactions. Memory is located neither in the hippocampus nor in the neocortex: the brain in its entirety as an information-processing system is just as involved in the emergence of memory as the whole organism (which is necessary for the functioning of the brain).

Of course it is plausible that these early experiences are then rewritten again and again and again, in later developmental phases.

In his theory of Neural Darwinism, Edelman (1992) illustrated this understanding of memory and remembering with the diagram shown in Figure 3.1, which he differentiates from the storehouse model and the memory models of classical cognitive science. He also contends that the neural network changes each time it produces memory—but it is always dependent on the "history" of the brain. Memory is thus seen as a constructive, adaptive process of the whole organism interacting with the environment, connecting knowledge gained by experience with analogous new situations; memory is part of the structure of the organism, which is changed by experience and reacts to new situations, such as an infection, in different ways—that is, memory is not stored in the brain. Thus, in contrast to "classical conceptualizations", the memory theories of "Embodied Cognitive Science" emphasize the *relevance, for the memory, of the interaction between the biological organism and its environment, the "embodiment", the "relatively inexact" but adaptive combination of new and earlier information.*

Regarding the above-mentioned controversial discussion, it is important that early interactions are stored in the body or in the

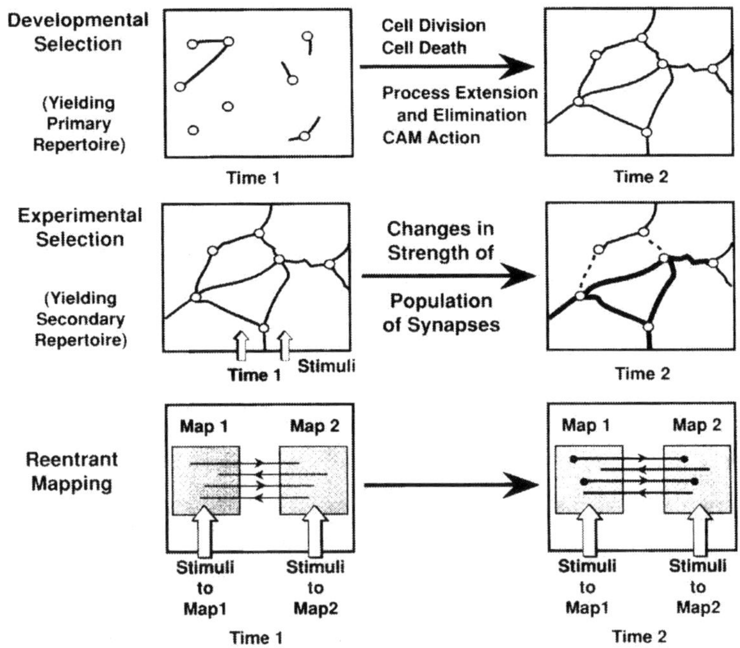

Figure 3.1. Parallel sampling of the environment by multiple sensory maps by a process of sensorimotor coordination—"reentrant mapping".

organism—that is, in the primary or secondary repertoire and neural maps, as Edelman calls them—and thus (dynamically unconsciously) determine the processing of new information.

Primary repertoire

The first connection of nerve cells—for example, those in the brain—is the result of a developmental selection taking place mainly during one's time as an embryo. Briefly, Edelman understands by this a selective process of a large number of neurons caused by genetic and social factors, because the primary cell processes of division, floating, death, adhesion, and induction do not only take place according to genetic conditions: they also differ according to time and place—that is, they are dependent on their location.

This means that from an initially immense surplus of nerve cells a tissue develops as a result of topobiological competition—in other words, cell floating and cell death, which look schematically like the one in the first line of graph 2. Edelman calls this network "primary repertoire". It forms the matrix of the nerve tissue of the brain. It forms the basis of a genetically controlled process that is subject to chemical influences and *thus the product of genetic make-up and environment—that is, an early interaction between the organism and the real world.* At this stage, there are as yet no working circuits, but there is a network capable of expansion.

Thus, this model suggests that very early experiences—such as Mr M's being with a depressed mother who then abandons him—influence the development of the primary neural network.

Secondary repertoire

This expansion requires the nerve cells' electric activity, the so-called *experimental selection,* in which the existing anatomy usually no longer changes. *Experimental selection* means that due to experience (behaviour), synaptic links in the existing population of synapses are selectively strengthened or weakened via specific biochemical processes. This mechanism, which selectively forms the basis of memory and a number of other functions, causes a variety of circuits (with strengthened synapses) in the anatomic network. The variety of these circuits forms the *secondary repertoire.*

Neural maps

The so-called neural maps develop from the functional circuits. They consist of some 10,000 neurons that functionally work in one direction. Each perceptive system—such as the visual system, the sensory surface of the skin, and so on—develops a variety of maps that are stimulated by impressions of different qualities: colour, touch, direction, temperature, and so forth. These maps are interconnected by parallel and reciprocal fabrics that enable a new and repetitive entry, run-through, and exchange of signals. If groups of neurons in a map are selected by stimuli, there is a simultaneous stimulation of the connected maps. With the renewed entry of impulses, the synapses in the neural groups of each map are strengthened or weakened, and the connections between the maps themselves are also modified.

This causes new, selective traits to emerge—in other words, there are "automatic" re-categorizations of current stimuli from different sensory channels. The organism makes sure that it has the ability to find its way in the interaction with the environment—that is, it compares current experiences with earlier ones by adapting the already known re-categorizations to a new situation after having received these new stimuli. This means that "categories" for the classification of current experiences (stimuli from different sensory channels) do not have to be defined "from the outside" but are formed "automatically", due to the topical sensorimotor coordination of the stimulated maps.

Edelman's main thesis is that—from the very beginning of conception—the neural network develops via an interaction of genetic and biological factors on the one hand and environmental influences on the other.

A central difference from the "classical theories of memory" is, thus—as already mentioned—the conceptualization of a dynamic and re-categorizing memory, which interacts with its environment as illustrated in Figure 3.1. Clancey (1991) gives the following definition of memory:

> Human memory is a capability to organize neurological processes into a configuration which relates perceptions to movements similar to how they have been coordinated in the past, [p. 253 (see also Edelman, 1992, p. 241; Leuzinger-Bohleber & Pfeifer, 2002)]

* * *

Back to our clinical case: From conception onwards, environmental experiences manifest themselves in the body, in the primary and secondary repertoire, in neural maps, and so on. The basic experience of patients like Mr M (and all the transvestite patients whom I have found in the psychoanalytical literature), that their male sex is not accepted by their mothers, has most probably been unconsciously engraved in the body. In this connection, we need more direct observations of the way mothers who cannot accept the sex of their baby boys touch their bodies, in particular their genitalia. (This is an example of the way conceptual research can initiate specific empirical research questions. Daniel Stern and others have published impressive studies on the interaction between depressed mothers and their infants. According to our clinical observation, we would like to test the hypothesis that depressed mothers who are unable to accept the sex of their baby boy will show not only the characteristics described by Stern, but some additional specific ones—for example, while cleaning the penis of their baby boys, and so on.)

The development of gender identity thus starts from the very beginning of life, not only during the oedipal phase, as postulated by Freud (as many contemporary authors have been discussing—see, e.g., Bohleber, 1982). The basic bodily experience of not being accepted by the (depressed) primary object with the sex that was given by nature is, as I see it now, the major unconscious source of transvestite gender development.

In this sense, we as psychoanalysts must be interested in the earliest "historical truths" that our patients experience in the particularly vulnerable first years of life. They are embodied (as Freud also pointed out, with his famous phrase that the ego was originally a physical one, a "body ego"). These early bodily sensations are—according to Freud's principle of "*Nachträglichkeit*"—reshaped again and again in response to subsequent experiences. It is therefore impossible to reconstruct them one-to-one on the one hand, but you always have to take into account the historical reality on the other.

* * *

To summarize: How could early object experiences with a depressed mother have affected Mr M's unconscious? Without discussing this question in detail here, I only postulate as follows:

1. In psychoanalytic terms, traces of early object experiences and the corresponding unconscious fantasies can be found in the—unconscious, sensorimotor, bodily—enactments of Mr M, and these become apparent mainly by processes of introjective and projective identification in the physical countertransference reactions of the analyst—for example, my intensive negative countertransference feeling in the initial interview, not being able to accept Mr M as "just as he is", feeling the impulse to send him away, into a sadistic treatment. Other examples are later sequences in which I—in analogy of a "dead mother"—felt like a dead "wax puppet" behind the couch, or "melted" with Mr M (analogously to one schema of being with a depressed primary object as described by Stern, 1995). These findings suggest that memory processes of traumatic childhood experiences can only

be detected by cautious observations of the enactment of the patient in the transference to the analyst.

2. According to the just outlined findings of Embodied Cognitive Science, these processes are based on sensorimotor-affective coordination processes: stimuli that (unconsciously) take up different stimuli in different sense organs in the current analytic situation (during the analytic session on the couch) are coordinated in the same way as in early pathogenic object relations. Although these sensorimotor coordination processes always result in ever new "constructions", due to the analogy to earlier situations they produce the same physical reactions (such as stomach aches) and feelings (of being absolutely alone, worthless, de-animated, dehumanized). Thus, "embodied" memories are constructed in the analytic relationship. They are not arbitrary but follow neural patterns that were acquired in earlier pathogenic object relations. Thus, the "historical truth" plays a decisive role for the process of recognition, even if it is placed in different narrative forms.

These findings of "Embodied Cognitive Science" illustrate, in my opinion, in a very precise way not only the important processes of introjective and projective identification but also why therapeutic changes do not occur after merely cognitive insights. In analogy to psychoanalytic–clinical experience, they are connected with remembering and working-through in the transference to the analyst.

This process of understanding is the step that follows the just outlined "embodied" observations in the transference/countertransference. To mention just one example: the myth of Narcissus, who fell fatally in love with his own face in the mirroring water, rejecting at the same time Echo, the nymph who really wanted to love him as an irreplaceable, unique object, was a valuable heuristic for me in order to conceptualize the preverbal, not yet symbolized bodily appeals of my patient and my own psychosomatic reactions, which were induced by him in images and eventually in verbal hypotheses. In this way I was presumably able to take on containing functions that Mr M had fundamentally lacked in his early object relations with his depressive and often even aggressively rejecting mother. I was able to offer Mr M images and verbal phrasings that would increasingly encode his own body language, the patient's biographic information on the dramatic birth, the severely depressed mother, the long separation during the second year of life after the death of the baby brother being, of course, indispensable for this. In this way we eventually succeeded in connecting Mr M's bodily reactions and most violent feelings towards the analyst—such as during the sequence planning his sex operation—with unconscious body fantasies and visualizations and verbalizations—that is, in initiating a symbolization of early, up to then unconscious bodily experiences. With his sex operation Mr M unconsciously planned to finally fulfil his mother's longing for a daughter, which was at the same time a definitive submission to her incapability to accept his male sex—as well as to revenge himself on her, destroying (in the transference) any libidinal cathexis of the object (see also the analogous discussion in interdisciplinary trauma research, e.g. Bohleber, 2000; Cooper, Kernberg, & Person, 1989; Laplanche, 1988; Laub, Peskin, & Auerhahn, 1995; Leuzinger-Bohleber, 2002; among others).

Summary

I have tried to illustrate here that clinical, conceptual, and empirical research in psychoanalysis have, since Freud's time, been in a continuous process of enlarging our knowledge about the unconscious fantasies and conflicts of our patients. It was a revolutionary insight, described by Freud a century ago, that perversions are connected with unsolved oedipal conflicts and an infantile compromise formation dealing with castration anxieties. Indeed—in the case of Mr M, the transvestite patient described here, and most of the cases reported in the clinical psychoanalytical literature so far—castration anxieties and an unsolved oedipal conflicts have been one unconscious source for a perverse development. In the 1980s many psychoanalytic theorists contended that severe unsolved conflicts during the individuation–separation phase (according to Margaret Mahler) presented an additional biographical and psychodynamic background for a transvestite symptom formation. As I discussed in this chapter, knowledge collected during recent decades by clinical researchers, empirical infant researchers, as well as by memory researchers in the field of the so-called Embodied Cognitive Science has added to a deeper and more precise understanding of the influence of the early object relations with a depressed mother. In the case of all the other transvestite patients whom I had found described in literature, the depressed mother had not been able to accept the sex of her baby boy. According to these studies, we can suppose that both maternal depression and her deep disappointment that the baby was not a girl might have influenced her bodily interaction with her infant. The unpleasant, unempathetic, and existential early interaction with the primary object must, according to my hypothesis, have been engraved in the body of the baby boy and influenced his gender development from the very beginning. The narcissistic defence ("narcissistic envelope") against an archaic form of unbearable depression, along with the development of a "false" (narcissistic) transvestite personality can be understood considering this biographical background. Mr M also seemed to be identified with the "dead mother", trying to revitalize her—for example, by the genital stimulation in the transvestite enactments. Thus, he was still unconsciously not individuated from the depressed, rejecting mother.

Commentary

Linda C. Mayes

Marianne Leuzinger-Bohleber has provided us with a number of potentially fruitful avenues for discussion. Her clinical material is very rich and intriguing, especially the layers of meaning that emerged one by one in her patient's understanding of his sexual orientation and conditions for sexual arousal. The material in her chapter is central to the theme of this book: the progression of theoretical models of sexuality since Freud's *Three Essays on the Theory of Sexuality* (1905d). She asks us to consider the material in at least two different ways: the first, surely, as a part of highlighting the theoretical shifts in understanding sexuality and especially the role of early attachments and object relations in defining the range and depth of sexual orientation. In her first perspective she presents us with a number of provocative hypotheses about the developmental precursors of her patient's sexual perversion; and especially she asks us to consider maternal depression as one of the precursors we must consider in sexual development. The second perspective she urges us to consider is how this kind of case material and other similar material can be used to inform the distinction she makes between conceptual and empirical research perspectives. Asking us to consider the translational efforts between the two approaches, she also asks how contemporary models of memory and learning at a neural level may be useful for our understanding of enduring patterns of behaviour and of personal narrative.

First, by way of the individual case material and the understanding of that material, let me highlight the metatheoretical levels that Leuzinger-Bohleber's hypotheses represent. There is the hypothesis that transvestism represents a defensive stance against the dangers of dependency: to be both man and woman, and especially not to need a mother or a woman for satisfaction and wholeness. At a similar developmental period, we might see transvestite organization as a response to separation–individuation: a solution that permits holding onto the mother always. A third is as a reaction to trauma—to maternal rejection, abuse, or hateful, destructive fantasies. In this case, Mr M's mother's severe postnatal depression was at least partly in reaction to his gender—she had wanted a girl, and she very expressly told him so. We might say that in his effort to understand his mother's mind as well as to ward off her destructive fantasies towards him, he adopts the gender she wants him to be.

Any one of these levels provides a coherent explanation for one aspect of the case material, raises possible hypotheses, and might suggest possible avenues for empirical approaches to follow up on these hypotheses. For example, we might propose that in situations in which postnatal maternal depression is experienced by the child as not just a passive withdrawal but also as actively hostile—in this instance, the mother expressly not wanting the child she has or with considerable negative attribution—there is more likely to be a negative developmental impact. We might also hypothesize that when the negative or hostile attributions relate to the child's gender, then the negative developmental impact may more likely be expressed in aspects of gender identity and the psychological conditions for sexual arousal. The empirical literature on the long-term developmental impact of maternal depression is very mixed surely in part because for individual dyads, the specific ways a depression is both expressed and experienced are salient—as both this case and these hypotheses potentially illustrate.

These kinds of hypotheses are examples of the very traditional model of how in-depth clinical work with an individual patient informs empirical approaches to larger groups of patients. Which brings me to Leuzinger-Bohleber's focus on conceptual–empirical research, a distinction she has written a great deal about. I shall surely defer to her expertise in this matter, but here are some additional questions to be considered.

(1) The underlying challenge of the conceptual–empirical distinction is that the interface of clinical and empirical endeavours broadly defines different epistemologies, different ways of knowing. Clinical perspectives, gathered one patient at a time at whatever level of clinical depth, are simply different ways of knowing, inasmuch as these typically emphasize individual characteristics and individual variation while minimizing commonalities, whereas empirical perspectives seek to find commonalties among individuals and minimize individual variation. How one epistemology informs the other is that one suggests hypotheses for the other—the clinical data from individuals may hint at possible fruitful lines of hypothesizing, while the empirical data from groups tests the relevancy of these hypotheses for patients that may share some common features and thus informs, in turn, the clinical work. Of course, how the empirical hypothesis testing informs individual clinical work depends in part on the relevancy of the particular set of common features for the clinical issue is question. So, for example, an empirical approach to sexual perversions might group together the various individual variations in conditions for arousal in ways that might inform developmental mechanisms, but this grouping would not necessarily be helpful in individual work with an individual patient.

(2) In developmental matters as complex as sexual orientation and the conditions for sexual arousal, can psychoanalytic data from individual patients serve to inform theories of causality? I would suggest that psychoanalytic data cannot inform studies of mechanism or causality in part exactly because psychoanalytic clinical data are gathered at such a close, individual level. As Leuzinger-Bohleber correctly suggests, it is very unlikely that any other clinical approach would have revealed the complexity of Mr M's developmental adaptation and sexual adjustment. On the other hand, data gathered at such a level of individual detail are often too close to inform an overall theory of developmental mechanism. When looked at up close, what may appear to be a contributing factor to transvestism, such as maternal depression raised in this particular case, may indeed be shared by many individuals and thus not be a specific causal pathway. Instead, such data may inform the individual clinician wanting to understand how he or she might approach another transvestite patient. The distinction is key—we may use the range of presenta-

tions from, for example, transvestite patients to inform the specificity of our treatment with them without any presumption that the issues most central to this group of patients in any way inform our theories of causality. So, for example, it may well be that separation–individuation concerns are uppermost in the material of many transvestite patients but this is not the same as a statement of causality. Rather it informs the therapist of the potential therapeutic landscape with such patients—a different emphasis.

(3) Making a distinction between conceptual and empirical research perhaps partially distracts us from an approach that psychoanalysts have made less use of: the qualitative/quantitative methods for taking advantage of single case studies. Data from our close-up clinical perspectives are especially suitable to these methods and present an opportunity that as a field we have taken advantage of in only a very few places.

(4) Finally, Leuzinger-Bohleber raises the implication of more recent work on learning and memory for how we think about narrative and reconstruction in psychoanalytic work. This is a very large topic, and it is important to be careful about reductionism regarding highly complex neurobiological models of learning at the neural level as these might be relevant to the psychological capacities of memory.

* * *

But I will close by underscoring the importance of Marianne Leuzinger-Bohleber's suggestion that early experiences in the care of another shape functional processes for handling stimulation and responding to levels of stress and emotional arousal—the specifics of the memories are less important than the functional systems that appear shaped by these early experiences. Preclinical work examining the intergenerational transmission of parenting behaviours has shown that not only are very specific patterns of parenting transmitted intergenerationally, but early parenting shapes later stress-regulatory capacities and curiosity/exploration: functional abilities shaped by early experiences.

4

The issue of homosexuality in psychoanalysis

Richard C. Friedman

Freud's views about sexuality provoked controversy, of course, and controversy stimulated by open discussion of human sexuality is still with us—even among psychoanalytic audiences!

I began research and scholarship in the area of human sexual orientation in the 1970s (Friedman, Green, & Spitzer, 1976; Friedman, Wollesen, & Tendler, 1976). During the three decades or so that I have presented talks in this area, I have found the intellectual atmosphere to be turbulent. Once, at a well-attended talk at a psychoanalytic association, an older man (I now qualify for that dubious distinction) interrupted my presentation by standing up and screaming: "You're wrong!! Don't you realize that homosexuality will lead to the end of civilization!!!" (He objected to my view that homosexuality is not inherently pathological.) On a number of occasions scheduled and publicized events by psychoanalytic associations—were suddenly cancelled on grounds that the topic of homosexuality was too controversial for discussion by psychoanalysts. After publication in 1994 of a special article on homosexuality in the *New England Journal of Medicine* (Friedman & Downey, 1994), Jennifer Downey and I received a fair amount of—what can only be described as hate—mail from health professionals . One editor of a major psychoanalytic journal told me—in the 1990s—that they were interested in my ideas about sex but would not consider any submission about homosexuality. What this meant was that there was no possibility of adequate peer review of this topic!

Defensive responses have not come exclusively from what I have come to term "the traditional psychoanalytic right wing" but soon came to include the "radical gay left" as well. For example, I recently chaired a national conference on homophobia for a major psychiatric association. A gay/activist psychiatrist/psychoanalyst who discusses homosexuality in the psychoanalytic literature was "outraged" that a "heterosexual" should lead such a discussion. He expressed this view openly and with the goal of setting precedent and establishing policy. These are only a few of the many incidents that have occurred over the years—including very recently—indicating how much conflict there is among psychoanalysts about homosexuality.

There is no discussing the issue of homosexuality in psychoanalysis without being aware of ideological influences on psychoanalytic thought, political correctness, bias, and prejudice—the latter sometimes denied and acted out. Of course, I have my own biases—we all do—and I will try to make these as transparent as possible along the way.

Many of the ideas that I discuss here have been initially discussed in some detail in my books on the subject: *Male Homosexuality* (1988) and, with Dr Jennifer Downey, *Sexual Orientation and Psychoanalysis* (Friedman & Downey, 2002).

Historical continuities and discontinuities

In the United States, at least through the 1970s, psychoanalysis generated the core ideas of psychiatry and, therefore, of all the mental health professions.

Psychoanalytic education stressed the necessity to preserve "traditions" of psychoanalysis generally, and at one's own psychoanalytic institute in particular. The traditions were more or less embodied in the belief systems of the training analysts. The beliefs of senior psychoanalysts, including training analysts, were by no means confined to psychoanalytic technique or the psychoanalytic clinical situation but included all aspects of human behaviour. I emphasize this because a radical dislocation occurred between the ideas about sexual orientation endorsed by the psychoanalytic establishment during the three decades following the Second World War, and subsequent psychoanalytic generations, in a way that was, I believe, unprecedented in the history of psychoanalysis—at least in the United States. Reverberations from this generational rift are still being experienced in organized psychoanalysis. The forces that led to this dislocation were born outside psychoanalysis, however, and did not originally emerge from within the psychoanalytic institutes.

During the three decades following the Second World War, psychoanalysts had more or less consistent systems of belief about sexuality and homosexuality—as they did about many other dimensions of behaviour (Bayer, 1981; Lewes, 1988; Wiedeman, 1962, 1974). If research had been carried out then on reliability of their core beliefs—about homosexuality—the measured inter-analyst agreement would probably have approached 100%. I strongly doubt that this would be the case today.

The DSM–III and homosexuality

In the process of creation of the DSM–III, American Psychiatry re-examined its evidence base (American Psychiatric Association, 1980). Organized psychiatry came into conflict with psychoanalysis around the twin issues of the nature of evidence and the nature of psychopathology. Influential analysts believed that knowledge of the unconscious was "special" and that it was not, and should not, be subject to usual academic standards of truth assessment. Some still believe this today.

By the time I began working with the DSM Committee, a decision had already been made to delete homosexuality from the diagnostic nomenclature; a decision with which I agreed. In rejecting the opinions of that time of the psychoanalytic establishment (who strongly urged that the diagnosis should be retained), the American Psychiatric Association also rejected the *method that the psychoanalytic community had adopted to assess the truth of its assertions.* This rejection occurred at the same time as the gay rights movement, which was expressed within psychiatry as well as the general society. The DSM Committee rejected the psychoanalytic perspectives of the time, however, not because of the influence of gay activism but, rather, because the database supporting key psychoanalytic inferences was flimsy. Interestingly, although there as been some improvement in this, the problem of a sparse database supporting psychoanalytic inferences about sexuality has by no means been solved.

Studies and case reports

When I reviewed the psychoanalytic literature on homosexuality in the mid-1970s for the DSM committee and in order to carry out my own research, I was astonished by how undisciplined and chaotic it was. Papers in major journals differed with respect to aspects of the patients' sexual histories, the presence of confounding major psychopathological syndromes, the specificity with which patients were discussed. The extra-analytic literature was rarely referred to. The psychoanalytic literature heavily emphasized male sexuality; the literature on female homosexuality was quite sparse in comparison (Friedman, 1988; Lewes, 1988; Wiedeman, 1962, 1974). In fact, in a 1998 article that Jennifer Downey and I published in *JAPA* (Downey & Friedman, 1998), we reported that the classical psychoanalytic literature contained only 68 cases discussing female homosexuality.

This notwithstanding, psychoanalysts made many assertions about homosexuality and bisexuality in men and women and usually disregarded the problem of selection bias.

As far as I could tell, there had only been one study of homosexuality carried out by practising psychoanalysts (Bieber et al., 1962).

Let me outline the few most important beliefs that analysts in the United States had about homosexuality when I began working in the field. Although most of those in the American community have changed their views, some have not—and some or all of these beliefs remain influential elsewhere in the world.

1. Homosexuality is pathological and results primarily from developmental derailment (during pre-oedipal and/or oedipal developmental phases).
2. All human beings are biologically predisposed to experience (positive) oedipal motives and conflicts. Resolution of these conflicts inevitably leads to heterosexuality.
3. The analytic process therefore, if successful, must result in heterosexuality.

4. Among patients—and nonpatients as well—homosexuality is evidence that the superego is impaired.
5. Among patients—and nonpatients as well—homosexuality is evidence of pathological cross-gendered identification (Friedman, 1988; Lewes, 1988; Socarides, 1978; Wiedeman, 1962, 1974).

Contemporary psychoanalytic issues–scientific/developmental

Let me change perspective at this point to the twenty-first century. Substantial attention has recently been devoted to the appropriate treatment of gay patients by psychoanalysts (Domenici & Lesser, 1995; Drescher, 1998; Duberman, 1991; Friedman, 1988; Friedman & Downey, 2004; Isay, 1989, 1996; Lewes, 1988; Phillips, 2003, 2004; Roughton, 1995a, 1995b). The issue of homosexuality should, however, not be framed as a "gay" issue: it must be viewed from a much wider perspective. It does not seem possible (to me) to think about "homosexuality", however this is defined, without thinking about "heterosexuality" and "bisexuality" as well. I think it important for psychoanalysts to endorse an open-minded, curious, and inquiring attitude about sexuality. In that regard, the "origins" of homosexuality, bisexuality, and heterosexuality—however these terms are defined—whether in individual people or groups, are and should be appropriate topics of inquiry for psychoanalysis. This perspective may be seen as politically incorrect by some who fear that such inquiry might further discriminate against non-heterosexual patients. I don't agree with this but recognize that such inquiry has to be approached with psychoanalytic sophistication. Exactly what "psychoanalytic sophistication" means is somewhat outside the scope of this chapter. It does not mean, however, that analysts should selectively investigate the underlying motives for homosexual desire in a gay patient, with the covert hope of helping her or him change sexual orientation.

Let me put forth some definitions. The term "homosexuality" does not refer to a unitary construct, and it is helpful to distinguish the dimensions of the term that refer to the erotic domain—sexual fantasy and activity—from those that refer to identity and social role. The term "gay", for example, refers to identity and/or social role (Friedman, 1988). I use the term "sexual fantasy" to refer to *consciously experienced* psychological imagery associated with feelings that are explicitly erotic and lustful and with physiological responses of sexual arousal (Friedman & Downey, 2002). The term "sexual orientation" refers to a person's potential to respond with sexual arousal or excitement (consciously experienced) to persons of the same gender, the opposite gender, or both (Friedman & Downey, 1994).

It has become apparent that both genes and *prenatal* hormones may influence the experience and activity of children and adults and, therefore, that the *time period* that psychoanalysts must consider in thinking about the origins of many behaviours in their patients has to be extended backwards—to begin with conception!

Genetic influences on sexual orientation

I will mention the area of genetics only briefly. An overview of this area reveals that the database is sparse, especially so with respect to women (Bailey & Benishay, 1993; Bailey, Dunne, & Martin, 2000; Bailey & Pillard, 1991; Bailey, Pillard, Neale, & Argei, 1993; Eckert, Bouchard, Bohlen, & Heston, 1986; Habel, 1950; Hamer, Hu, Magnuson, Hu, & Pattatucci, 1993; Kallman, 1952a, 1952b; Kendler, Thornton, Gilman, & Kessler, 2000; Rice, Anderson, Risch, & Ebers, 1995; A. R. Sanders, 1998; J. Sanders, 1934; Whitam, Diamond, & Martin, 1993). The major research question seems to be whether there are genetic influences on homosexuality. An idea that I have heard bandied about in some psychoanalytic circles is that "homosexuality is genetic". Here the term "genetics" seems to be used in a metaphorical sense—to mean innate and unchangeable. That, of course, is reductionistic and not data-based. The behavioural genetic literature is quite relevant for psychoanalysis, however, and genetic influences on homosexual orientation—at least in men—seem to be important in subgroups.

Sexual differentiation of the brain

Whereas the area of behavioural genetics can be compartmentalized by psychoanalytic clinicians to some degree, the area of sexual differentiation of the brain cannot. By "compartmentalization" what I mean is an attitude that a friend and training analyst expressed when he told me: "At some point I'll catch up with the genetic issues—but, frankly, what difference does it make in my analytic work with patients? I don't try to change anyone's sexual orientation—genetics is not really relevant to office practice!"

Although I don't share the view that advances in knowledge relevant to our field should be thought of as "specialized" and split off from it, I do understand what my colleague meant. The area of sexual differentiation of the brain, however, is fundamentally different from the area of behavioural genetics. It is not possible to think adequately about erotic desire and activity, gender identity/gender role, or gender differences in behaviour without being aware that sexual differentiation of the brain occurs and being cognizant of its behavioural manifestations (Breedlove, 1994; Gorski, 1991; Hines, 1998; McEwen, 1983). Relevance of the area of sexual differentiation of the brain extends well beyond the specific question: "Are there prenatal hormonal influences on *sexual orientation?*" Knowledge of this area is necessary to adequately understand the way children experience and express gender-role behaviour (Diamond, 1982, 1997; Diamond & Sigmundson, 1997). This is particularly important for understanding clinical issues in nonheterosexual patients.

Gender-role behaviour, childhood play, and peer relationships

Thinking about human sexuality from a developmental perspective requires us to attend to many areas—attachment behaviour, gender identity development, familial relationships, cognitive development, to name just a few. I have chosen the area of gender-role behaviour to discuss more fully here because it bridges the gap, to some degree, between scientific/developmental and clinical issues. Because of space constraints, my emphasis is more on males than females.

It is now apparent that important gender differences in behaviour are attributable to sexual differentiation of the brain (Friedman, Richart, & Vande Wiele, 1974; Maccoby, 1998; Maccoby & Jacklin, 1974). I note this with some anxiety because this area is a minefield, as was recently discovered by the President of Harvard University.

Probably the gender difference most extensively documented to date is in play behaviour—primarily so-called "rough-and-tumble play" (RTP) (Maccoby, 1998; Maccoby & Jacklin, 1974; Meaney, 1989; Meaney, Stewart, & Beatty, 1985; Pelligrini & Smith, 1998). Boys and girls play differently (Thorne, 1993), and some of their differences are attributable to the influences of prenatal testosterone on brain embryogenesis. The differences result in behavioural interactions and cascades, leading to mid- and late-childhood *gender-segregated play*. This is a phenomenon that occurs across cultures, is associated with different gender-role fantasies experienced by boys and girls, and, as I mentioned, has great relevance for understanding clinical work with all patients but particularly nonheterosexual patients. The notion of "biological influence" on mid, and late, childhood play and peer behaviour does not exclude the importance of influences of caretakers and assumes ongoing shaping of behaviour by experience and fantasy to some degree.

In thinking about gender differences in play, it is helpful to have two different behavioural models in mind. One is the behaviour found among large groups. The second is the fantasy and activity found among individuals. Individuals fall along a distribution spectrum with regard to "rough-and-tumble play", for example. If one measures the behaviours quantitatively, the "statistical means"—no matter how parameters are defined—for boys and girls differ, but the curves overlap. Some boys are not strongly predisposed to RTP, and some girls are. The predisposition of a particular individual, however, may well be "set" as part of her or his constitutional predisposition.

Temperamental differences within genders

The notion of a spectrum for expressivity of androgen effects on post-natal behaviour is useful for understanding temperamental differences *within genders*. It is helpful, for example, to think of boys as falling along a spectrum in the degree to which they are drawn towards rough-and-tumble activities (RTP) and prototypical boyhood aggressivity. Among boys, on the more extreme end of the spectrum, the innate tendency is strong and may be likened to a white-water stream. Parents—and teachers—must be creative in attempting to cope with it, and I have seen many in consultation who are anxious about being swept away. Many boys fall in the middle part of the spectrum, and some boys seem not to evince much behavioural evidence of the androgen effect.

Childhood RTP is an important part of a behavioural cluster, including preference for stereotypical cross-gender activities (such as playing "house", for example), for having a girl as "best friend" during mid and late childhood, and playing predominately with girls (Bailey & Zucker, 1995; Zucker & Bradley, 1995).

Temperament, gender-role behaviour, and sexual orientation

It has been established that patterns of childhood cross-gender sex-typed behaviour are different between gay and heterosexual populations.

For example, Bailey and Zucker reviewed all studies published in English in which homosexual and heterosexual individuals were queried about their childhood cross-gender-typical interests and activities. Thousands of subjects were reported on. In every study, regardless of when it was published, method of sample selection, or research design, childhood gender role was recalled by homosexuals as more atypical with regard to sex-stereotypic behaviour than by heterosexuals (Bailey & Zucker, 1995).

I mentioned earlier that sex-segregated play tends to occur during mid and late childhood and the behaviour of children in sex-segregated groups is different—asymmetrical. Boys' peer groups tend to be larger, more hierarchically organized, more aggressive, and much less tolerant of cross-gender behaviour than those of girls.

In free play groups boys often tend to devalue behaviours labelled feminine and to label behaviours feminine that they devalue (Fine, 1987). Juvenile boys—and usually not girls—derisively label others "fag", for example, and bully them. Atypical gender-role behaviour may also trigger aggressive behaviour in adult males—including fathers. Boys on a gay developmental track are more likely than those on a heterosexual track to be bullied by other boys and men—sometimes including their fathers—because of what I will term here their gender-role temperaments. Because all male groups of juveniles are often "walled off" from adults, aggression among children may occur without adult awareness.

Let me pull together a few major points here.

- Most gay men have been bullied, threatened, menaced, or assaulted (by males).
- The time period when such interactions usually begin is often late childhood. They occur later as well, however.

- Such interactions may be repetitive and so severe that they induce traumatic/stress responses.
- Such responses may occur among nonheterosexual patients whose earlier lives within their families may have been stable and loving. Psychopathology in this group may be primarily a reaction to trauma.

I would like to elaborate on this a bit. Because clinical psychoanalysts lean heavily on paradigms of psychopathology emphasizing pre-oedipal and oedipal phase internalizations, psychoanalysts tend to be strongly aware of *intra-familial* determinants of psychopathology. In my clinical work with gay patients, however, I have seen many in whom symptoms appear primarily to result from late childhood trauma. The key psychosocial problems seem to occur when the child moves out of the family and into the world of peers. Here some of these children encounter brutality for the first time, and the consequences may be damaging.

The complexity of this area is increased because traumatic responses may occur among a different group of nonheterosexual patients who do come from familial environments of neglect and/or abuse and who have antecedent psychopathology. Additive complex psychopathological combinations may then occur. Thus, a child analyst, for example, may encounter patients with abundant oedipal and pre-oedipal pathology who also become brutalized by peers later on.

Male aggression triggered by atypical gender-role behaviour

The tendency of some males to respond to atypical gender-role behaviour with aggression must be understood within the context of male aggression generally. The fact that in all societies throughout recorded history human males have always been more aggressive than females no matter how aggression has been defined is but one piece of evidence indicating biological influences on male aggression (Friedman, Richart, & Vande Wiele, 1974; Moyer, 1976). Sexual differentiation of the brain is one such important influence. Similarities between the aggressive behaviour of human males and of our close mammalian relatives suggests genetic influences as well.

Homosexuality and childhood gender-role behaviour

The determinants of the association between childhood gender-role temperament and adult sexual orientation remain to be established. Since the association is so robust and has been reported among patients and nonpatients, some type of biological influence seems likely. Such influence probably involves sexual differentiation of the brain, although intermediate pathways remain to be established. Since many boys with the same type of temperament as those on a gay developmental track become heterosexual, a simple "cause–effect" biological model does not seem likely.

Plasticity of the erotic image

The notion of behavioural plasticity is psychoanalytically friendly. Clinical psychoanalysts have been enthusiastic about the good news that psychotherapy can change the brain, for example (Kandel, 1999). Our field has been somewhat cooler, I think, towards the notion that there are some attributes of mind that do not appear to be plastic and that these limit what analysts can seek to accomplish. One area that has attracted attention with regard to plasticity is the degree to which the erotic image is changeable.

The image associated with erotic arousal/excitement is part of an internally experienced erotic narrative (Person, 1995; Stoller, 1975a, 1975b, 1979b). The onset of consciously experienced erotic fantasies tends to occur among males during childhood and early adolescence (Herdt & McClintock, 2000). These fantasies, which occur during masturbation and in response to many stimuli of daily life and are mobilized by pornography, are inclusive but also exclusive. For many but not all men, once these fantasies are in place they tend to remain more or less constant for life. Women—far more diverse in many dimensions of their sexual experience and activity—are more likely to manifest plasticity with respect to their sexual fantasies and activity (Baumeister, 2000). Thus, women may experience novel homosexual fantasies relatively late in life, often associated with meaningful and intense emotional attachments (Downey & Friedman, 1998). The innately determined lack of plasticity among most men with respect to the erotic object may explain why so many gay patients in generations past could not alter their sexual orientation during analysis, despite loving relationships with women and despite their own energetic attempts to do so and those of their analysts. Because *some* men are probably more malleable than *most* in this respect, great caution must be exercised about generalizing from a particular analyst's experiences with a particular patient in this regard.

Clinical issues: introduction

Patients in the twenty-first century are not like those in the nineteenth (with some dramatic exceptions, of course). For example, I am analysing a man who has been HIV+ for more than 20 years, and another became HIV+ during treatment. These days, patients of every sexual orientation meet in Internet chat-rooms. One of my patients has put a nude picture of himself with an erect penis on the net, another periodically threatens that he will go to pornographic sites involving children. (As it happens, this patient is gay; however, the same threat could obviously have been made by a heterosexual patient.) Gay male colleagues and friends are at present in the process of adopting a child conceived by a surrogate mother. One of my gay patients has married another man (in a state that endorses gay marriage). His homophobic mother attended the ceremony—providing much useful material for analytic work. Another—a middle-aged man from the Midwestern United States—was not allowed to speak at the funeral of his father because he is gay. His brother and sister each delivered funeral orations.

Diagnostic issue

When it comes to diagnosis of psychopathology in relation to sexual orientation, the issues are quite complex, and no one really has the last word on the matter.

By the 1980s it had become apparent that some type of multiaxial diagnostic schema had to be used by psychoanalysts. Prior to the acceptance of multiaxial diagnosis by analysts, a simple linear model was popular in which "very early"—such as preoedipal—traumata were hypothesized to "cause" very severe psychopathology.

Some theorists hypothesized that homosexuality was "caused" by such traumata. Abandonment of that model is in keeping with in advances in science and in descriptive psychiatry as well.

I find it useful to distinguish the type of character defences used by a particular patient from his level of ego integration. Sexual orientation then becomes a third descriptive feature of someone's "profile", as it were. A homoerotic image may be experienced totally or partially (along with a heteroerotic image) by patients who are well integrated as well as those who are integrated at a borderline level (Friedman, 1998). Men at the lower level of ego integration are prone to become involved in impulsive/compulsive sexual activities that are often associated with substance abuse and are often "unsafe". These men may be gay, bisexual, or heterosexual. I emphasize this because a commonly held prejudicial belief about gay men is that they are "promiscuous". This attribution is incorrect, although it is likely that gender differences being what they are, women may exert a "braking effect" on the sexual activities of many heterosexual men.

Homophobia

Homophobia and internalized homophobia

The psychoanalytic community is indebted to extra-psychoanalytic psychologists who introduced the topics of homophobia and internalized homophobia into the clinical literature (Malyon, 1982; Weinberg, 1972). Of course, the term "homophobia" is not really accurate from an analytic perspective. So-called homophobic people are usually not "phobic" in a technical sense. I use it because the term has entered general usage. "Internalized homophobia" may occur in patients who are truly gay and those who are bisexual.

Internalized homophobia in gay patients

We have no specific paradigm that explains in a simple unitary way why some men are more or less totally homosexual in their consciously experienced erotic lives, some are bisexual, and others are heterosexual. Combinations of genetic, neuroendocrine, and experiential factors presumably interact differently to influence the three major outcomes. Hopefully psychoanalysts will be part of teams that shed light on this area.

In thinking about psychopathology, let me first consider patients who are truly gay.

One major psychopathological "issue" in these patients—I think the most important large "issue"—concerns their negative internalizations. Psychoanalysis has already made important contributions in understanding this area and will, I am confident, continue to do so in the future. The extensive experience we have had with the area of internalization generally serves us well here.

One basic psychoanalytic concept that I find particularly useful is that of condensation. I use the term in a somewhat different way, however, from Freud's original usage of it. What I mean is conflation of multiple aspects of psychological functioning occurring over extended time periods. These conflations involve fantasies, conscious and unconscious, leading to a final common pathway: negative labelling of the self, triggered by awareness of—in Isay's terms—"being homosexual" in some sense.

Let me outline some conflations that I have found clinically important.

First and probably most important is identification with multiple aggressors. Conflation of fantasies from different developmental phases occurs here. For example, someone who has been bullied by peers may conflate fantasies generated in response to those stimulated by abusive behaviour from his father. As well we know, imagery of the father may in fact be the outer layer of deeper imagery involving the mother. These images may have—in traditional terms—oedipal and pre-oedipal components and influences.

Imagery of the gender-valued self-representation may become conflated with erotic imagery. Thus an awareness of being unworthy and inadequate—associated with feelings of guilt and shame—may have gender-valued components (e.g. "I don't fit into groups of other boys. I am unmasculine and inadequate") and erotic components (e.g. "I am a bad person because I have been sexually attracted to my father").

Other conflations typically involve fantasies generated in response to internal and psychosocial environments that do not primarily and fundamentally concern "sexual orientation" but, rather, have to do with other issues (stress between the parents and divorce leading to depression, for example). The developing child attributes all "bad" feelings to his sexual orientation. By the time he is an adult and on our couch, he has woven what seems to him to be a seamless narrative "explaining" his suffering in terms of his "homosexuality".

In considering psychoanalytic work with adults, it is helpful to attempt to separate the different levels of fantasy about self and others that lead to a final common pathway. In that regard, it is helpful to distinguish the homoerotic image itself from other aspects of the self representation that may seem chronic but are likely to be malleable. The notion of malleability brings us back to the area of the erotic image. In the men I am discussing here, the erotic image itself does not appear to be malleable and in itself is not a response to unconscious anxiety. The "shape and colouring" of the erotic image is another matter, however. Certain of its features—such as situations associated with or generating sexual desire, aspects of the sexual scenario—may change during treatment. In saying this I am relying on clinical knowledge and not on published studies. Successful treatment, however, seems—at least in my experience—to be associated with a movement away from dehumanized sadistic/masochistic scenarios that are experienced in a rigid and limiting way and towards some type of authentic human interaction.

Because of the way psychoanalysts tend to think about sexual orientation today has shifted so much, our field has not had time to adequately consider the myriad transference and countertransference issues relevant to work with the patients I discuss here. Space does not allow me to discuss transference, but I do want to touch here on the issue of countertransference.

A countertransference problem that used to be common—now less so, I think—was the analyst's desire to "rescue" his /her patient from a "gay life style" and steer him towards conventional heterosexual marriage. Analysts also struggled with the notion that values and attitudes of gay men about their sexuality are different from the conventional heterosexual model.

As more heterosexual psychoanalysts became "gay-friendly", I think our field has changed the way we tend to think about the different combinations of "recreational–procreational and relational" motives for sexual activity. We have moved, I think, towards relativism, and we are less likely to be provoked to abandon our helpful analytic attitudes that have served us in good stead with so many other patients.

Gay analysts, however, may have countertransference problems with non-heterosexual patients as well. Many have experienced anti-homosexual prejudice from heterosexuals during their lives. Some have had painful experiences with heterosexual analysts, which have led to unresolved conflicts. Of course, these problems may also be experienced and expressed in analytic work with heterosexual patients.

Bisexuality

Bisexuality remains what I might term an island of confusion in an ocean of progress in analytic thought about sexual orientation (Friedman & Downey, 2002). Is bisexuality (as we understand it today) inherently pathological?

How do we conceptualize bisexuality as opposed to homosexuality or heterosexuality?

Some meaningful degree of bisexuality among men is probably reasonably common (Laumann, Gagnon, Michael, & Michaels, 1994; McConaghy, 1993). There is no social niche for so-called "bisexuals"—no real subculture that supports their psychosocial integration the way the gay subculture does for so many gay males. Some men who are bisexual with respect to sexual fantasy and activity consider themselves gay, some consider themselves heterosexual; a relative few, I think, consider themselves neither. This, of course, leads to confusion in designing research studies. Many studies group bisexuals with homosexuals, for example—men who have sex with men. Some that use self-labelling as criteria for assignment to categories will place someone into a heterosexual group because he labels himself so, no matter what his sexual behaviour. Of course, some bisexual people change their sexual identity labelling over time.

I doubt that the determinants of bisexuality are correlated with innate determinants of any type of psychopathology. Indeed, one way of thinking about bisexuality is that it provides more opportunities for experience and for growth than might be the case among those in whom options are more limited.

Our patients who are bisexual do tend, however, to present interwoven strands in which bisexuality is connected to their psychopathology, and it is here that I now turn.

Social factors during the entire life cycle of the patient are usually negatively biased towards homosexuality. The condensations discussed earlier for gay patients may selectively apply to the homoerotic component of hetero-homoerotic imagery. Lifetime exposure to sexism and heterosexism, by peers and authority figures—not to mention developmental experiences with organized religions—may all have their effects.

Let me discuss the erotic image in bisexual men—with the qualification that my thoughts are conjectural. Clinical experience suggests that one has to think about erotic imagery in bisexual men somewhat differently than in those at either end of the homosexuality–heterosexuality spectrum. Both components of bisexual imagery—the hetero- and the homoerotic image—are likely to be more malleable and less fixed in many bisexual men in ways that are different from those in truly gay or heterosexual men. Either may be amplified or suppressed/repressed. This may be anxiety-provoking for therapists because we are, I think, all more comfortable with unitary models that seem to explain everything.

Borderline bisexual patients

Returning to the distinction between the erotic components of psychological functioning and the identity/role components, it can readily be seen that borderline bisexual patients have particularly difficult adaptational problems (Friedman, 1988).

I don't believe that bisexuality is more common among borderline patients or that there is any inherent connection between the two. Borderline bisexual patients are not uncommon, however, and these patients have lured many an analyst into the countertransference error of attempting to directly answer their question "Am I gay or heterosexual?" Here the patient formulates a simple question/answer format about his sexual orientation in an attempt to solve a pervasive identity problem. Identity diffusion persists, of course, no matter what the answer to the question is. Answers such as "you are truly gay" or "you are basically heterosexual" tend to limit the analyst's options to work therapeutically with the underlying conflicts influencing the identity diffusion.

CONCLUSION

In the twenty-first century our sometimes beleaguered discipline faces the challenge of making many types of integrations.

At the basic science level, psychoanalysts are increasingly working with neurobiologists and other extra-analytic investigators in interdisciplinary teams. This notwithstanding, I think that there is still a culture gap between the attitudes and values of researchers and those of many clinical practitioners.

Understanding human sexuality today requires an informed attitude about knowledge coming from extra-analytic sources, including neurobiology. A special problem exists in the relationship between psychoanalysis and psychobiology, I suspect because analytic candidates and even senior faculty at institutes vary in their knowledge of and attitudes towards biology. The "new biology", however, makes it clear that "psychobiology" should no longer be equated with drive theory. Childhood play, for example, is as rooted in psychobiology as adult sexuality and aggression. I think that the earliest maternal–child relationship is so rooted as well (Mayes, 2005). Reframing psychoanalytic attitudes towards psychobiology remains, of course, a pedagogical problem in our field.

We analysts find it difficult to abandon ideas that may have outlived their usefulness but may generate the fondness that we feel for familial traditions. In that regard, the analytic experience with homosexuality led Jennifer Downey and me to pose revision in the way that psychoanalysts conceptualize the Oedipus complex.

> We conjecture that the aggressive component of oedipal themes is much more prevalent than the erotic component and that the competitive–aggressive motivations of oedipal aged boys do not occur as a consequence of sexual desires for the mother. Rather they are experienced and expressed as a result of the influence of prenatal androgens on the brain. [Friedman & Downey, 1995a]

Space constraints do not allow me to comment on this further here, however. This was but one of a number of fundamental revisions that (we felt) psychoanalysis should make in response to incoming knowledge.

This includes revision in the way we think about the development and psychological functioning of the genders. Psychoanalysis has to struggle to get clarity about the aspects of psychological functioning that men and women share and those that seem more gender-specific. If the brains of females and males are different in certain respects yet similar in others, is it not possible that unconscious mental processes in females and males might prove different in certain respects, yet similar in others? Psychoanalytically informed research comparing gay men to lesbians may be of assistance in clarifying issues here.

With respect to erotic sexuality we can, I think, greatly contribute to knowledge about the degree of plasticity vs. rigidity of the erotic object/situation. How much does erotic fantasy/activity change during psychoanalytic work? Posing the question about all patients, not just those who are nonheterosexual, directs attention to the need for descriptive history about sexual experience and activity among our patients. Pooling data about this area—particularly data acquired longitudinally during and following treatment—will be of great value.

In conclusion, the homosexuality issue directs our attention to the influence of *bias* on psychoanalytic thought. Many different biases have exerted and sometimes continue to exert additive effects. Of these, arguably the most important has been the antiscientific attitude that dominated the field for many years. This resulted in inadequate methodological protection against such biases as sexism and heterosexism influencing the belief system of many analysts. An early example of the deleterious consequences of this was the widespread acceptance by psychoanalysis for many years of the so-called "clitoral–vaginal transfer theory" of female psychosexual development. Correction of this erroneous concept began as a result of the extra-analytic research of Masters and Johnson (1966).

Although increasing attention has been devoted to the need to integrate psychoanalytic knowledge with that of other fields, many problems still remain to be addressed. The issues raised by homosexuality may be seen as a case example of general problems still requiring creative adaptation by our field.

Commentary

Anne-Marie Sandler

The topic of homosexuality is so vast and the various points taken up in Friedman's chapter so complex, that I thought the best use I could make of the space at my disposal was to limit myself to a few personal comments.

When a German-speaking friend of mine heard that I had been asked to discuss work on this topic, she sent me a copy of a letter that Freud is supposed to have written to the mother of a homosexual. It reads:

> *I take it from your letter that your son is a homosexual. I was strongly impressed by the fact that in your comments about him you do not use this word. May I ask you why you are avoiding it? Homosexuality is certainly of no advantage but it is not something of which one needs to be ashamed; it is no vice, no degradation and it cannot be described as an illness. We consider it as a deviation of the sexual function caused by a certain cessation (stoppage) of the sexual development. Many greatly respected people, in old and present times, have been homosexuals, among them many of the greatest men (Plato, Michelangelo, Leonardo da Vinci, et cetera). It is a great injustice and a cruelty to consider homosexuality as a crime. . . .*

Despite these words of Freud, we all know how homosexuals were thought of in the not-so-distant past as depraved and unstable individuals, dangerous to society. Gradually, over the last 50 years, this view of homosexuality has been challenged, and some strata of public opinion have taken a more liberal view. There is no doubt that nowadays most people reject wholeheartedly the idea of criminalizing homosexuality and more people accept that the homosexual individual has a specific way of relating, no longer deviant, debased, or perverse, but different. However, it seems to me that we need to understand more deeply why many heterosexual men continue to react to homosexual men with strong hostility and deep contempt, especially if the homosexual has an openly feminine attitude and appears camp. Such clear disapproval and rejection does not seem so evident in the case of heterosexual women faced with homosexual female individuals.

I feel that it is important to reflect on the way the whole issue of homosexuality has become politicized and how emotions run high both on the part of the conservative so-called moral opponents to the idea of the normality of homosexuality as well as on the part of the gay and lesbian groups who insist that only they can speak on the topic. As we heard from Richard Friedman, this makes research in this area very difficult and challenging, as one can find oneself so easily in the middle of the most passionate and emotional debate, which makes reasoned thinking almost impossible.

Even though Freud and the psychoanalysts after him have studied the central importance and the complexity of sexuality in the life of individuals, there is still a lot that we do not fully comprehend. This particularly applies to the area of object choice, of the balance between lust and love in different individuals, and the factors that allow some couples to maintain their sexual excitement and gratification throughout their union while others do not, as well as the complex relation between aggression and love in the economics of a gratifying sexual act. The same complexity exists in the field of homosexuality. I am somewhat sorry that Friedman does not refer to the fact that we are really always dealing with a spectrum of homosexualities, not simply one homosexuality that covers all homosexual behaviour. It seems to me necessary to conceive of a broad field, which would include a great variety of sexual behaviour, from the normal to the pathological, both for the heterosexual and for the homosexual.

We have all heard of, and some of us have treated, homosexual men whose sexual excitement and gratification is linked with nightly "cottaging" in order to find an unknown partner for a one-night stand. In these encounters one could say that the other, the object, seems valued because of its total non-existence, its complete anonymity. The excitement and the gratification of the sexual act appears restricted to the genitalia, not to a whole person. I have never met lesbians who engage systematically in one-night stands in the same way as some homosexual men do. This rather compulsive behaviour must be contrasted with homosexual individuals who establish important homosexual relationships, often with a father/son feel or a privileged/underprivileged quality. These relationships can last for many years or even, on occasion, for a lifetime. Not infrequently they may have a feel of sadomasochistic interaction, but this may not be central to the relationship. In my limited clinical experience with this group of homosexual men and women I have become very aware of the frequent presence of a powerful source of anxiety, centred very often around painful jealousy, fear of abandonment, and preoccupation with ageing. To these two contrasting groups, we must also add an important group of homosexuals who have been abused in childhood, often for a prolonged period, and who in turn become abusers. Questions have to be asked, of course, whether there could be some unconscious elements that make some children more vulnerable to abuse than others, as we know that not all children in care or in dangerously promiscuous environments are abused. This is a very delicate and complex area of necessary research. It also seems to me to raise the age-old question of how much the environment can influence the role of the genes and of the prenatal hormones.

I was very interested in what Friedman had to say about the plasticity of the erotic imagery in the homosexual man or woman. He uses the term "sexual fantasy" to refer to consciously experienced psychological imagery associated with feelings that are explicitly erotic and lustful and are accompanied by physiological responses of sexual arousal. According to him the onset of consciously experienced erotic fantasies tends to occur during childhood and early adolescence in boys. It is masturbation, the many stimuli of daily life, and pornography that produce these fantasies, and for many men these will remain more or less constant for life. It is interesting to note that this is different for women, who are more likely to show plasticity in respect to their sexual fantasies. This confirms the position of Moses and Eglé Laufer towards homosexuality in men. They viewed adolescence as the period during which the male individual's sexual orientation is sealed.

Although I absolutely agree that psychoanalytic treatment of homosexuals must not aim to alter the patient's sexual orientation, it does seems important to allow them to express and face their internal malaise. Even though today a homosexual is no longer prosecuted or a pariah of society and may possibly marry and even have children, the reality remains that he cannot take part, together with his partner, in the act of reproduction. Sexuality and intercourse may remain exciting and pleasurable, but the experience that intercourse with a loving other can be an act of wondrous creativity is denied to them. I imagine that some people would call me homophobic because of these statements, yet I do think that this limitation in homosexual encounters is of importance.

I do not think that we ought to deny that to be a homosexual is often very difficult and is frequently, if not always, accompanied by considerable feelings of shame. Even though public reaction is slowly changing, homosexuality is still often met with a gut feeling of rejection and disgust. During adolescence, if not earlier, even the more protected homosexuals will have faced repeated rebuke, humiliating remarks, endless mocking, and isolation. Most of the homosexual patients I have treated suffered from painfully poor self-esteem. They had felt excluded from the normal social life of their peers and often sensed the disappointment and estrangement in their parents, teachers, and colleagues. I do not think that one can explain this simply by recognizing that males are more aggressive than females. This does not deny that on the whole lesbians appear to be less openly victimized than are male homosexuals.

In psychoanalysis, the importance of the countertransference is paramount. In an effort to be in tune with one's homosexual or lesbian patients, the analyst may, on the one hand, be afraid of appearing or of being homophobic and on the other hand may feel inhibited from relying on his or her heterosexual inner experiences. Both these difficulties can lead to something stilted in the relationship. This, in turn, is often picked up by the homosexual patients, who tend to be particularly sensitive to the nature and the quality of the relationship.

Friedman gives a useful list of the most important beliefs held by psychoanalysts in the 1970s. These reflect the view that homosexuality is pathological and the result of a developmental derailment early in life and certainly during the pre-oedipal and oedipal phases. Evidence of pathological identification—that is, of cross-gender identification—confounded this view. Analysts believed that all human beings were biologically predisposed to experience positive oedipal conflicts and that thus their resolution would lead inevitably to heterosexuality. With these convictions, it was naturally thought that a successful analysis of a homosexual patient would result in a change of orientation. It seems to me important to recognize that there are some homosexuals who embark on an analytic treatment in the hope of being helped to become heterosexuals and others who feel satisfied with their sexual orientation but wish to get help for a series of distressing symptoms.

The important question for psychoanalysts who are treating patients of the first group is to discover whether the distress is linked to painful fantasies that they associate with homosexuality—for example shame, fear of rejection, and contempt from others, or whether homosexual relationships are used defensively by a person who has heterosexual wishes, fantasies, and longings towards members of the opposite sex. In such a case the turning to homosexuality could be transient, as can sometimes be the case in adolescence, and the homosexual longings disappear when the anxiety linked, for example, to violence or to terrifying fantasies about the vagina or the penis is analysed. The aim of analysis in both cases is to reduce anxiety and explore the unconscious fantasies concerning the body and sexuality. I believe that we would nowadays understand the attempts of a psychoanalyst to influence a patient's sexual orientation as a countertransference enactment that ought to have been contained and worked through by the analyst.

5

Developmental research on childhood gender identity disorder

Susan Coates

Children with childhood gender identity disorder (CGID) are obsessed with the wish to be the other gender. One 3-year-old expressed it clearly: "I hate myself. I don't want to be me. I want to be someone else. I want to be a girl."

The problems with gender identity that I am interested in are those in which gender is recruited to solve unresolved issues of trauma in the parental generation, where unconscious anxieties over power and/or abuse have haunted parents and where these issues have become represented in the parental mind in gender preoccupations. In effect, the child's mind is recruited to solve these problems for the parents, but at great cost to the child in terms of his or her own autonomy and authenticity. The boy with extreme cross-gender identification is perceived by the parent as sweet, adorable, and loving and, in the parent's mind, unlike other boys, whom they perceive to be aggressive and destructive and who would have the potential to be triggers to their often unbearable memories of psychological misuse.

A child's sense of her or his own gender emerges in a very complex matrix that offers many surprises to the careful observer.

The child's conception of gender

The construction of the child's sense of gender begins by the second half of the first year of life. Between 6 and 12 months babies look more at same-sex pictures than at other-sex pictures (Lewis & Brooks-Gunn, 1979). When presented with anatomically correct dolls, infants can identify which doll they look like by age 2 (de Marneffe, 1997). In reference to the latter, however, if you ask the question in a different way—for example, by presenting a picture of a nude boy and a nude girl and asking which one is a boy and which one is a girl—you might be surprised to discover that many 2-year-old children will look at you oddly, as if you got it wrong, and say with some degree of indignity: "I can't tell which one is a boy or a girl, because they don't have their clothes on." At this age children know which doll they look like, but their construction of the categories of "boy" and "girl" is highly concrete and is determined by external characteristics, such as clothes and hair length, not by anatomical sex. By age 2, as language comes on line, children can use the verbal label "boy" or "girl" correctly when referring to adults, and within 6 months, by age 2½, they can do the same with peers and with themselves (Fagot, 1985). Remarkably, by age 5 more than half of all children still do not understand the defining role of genitalia in establishing sex categorization (Bem, 1989). This occurs even in children who can tell you that girls have vaginas and boys have penises. For example, one 3-year-old, who knew that boys have penises and girls have vaginas, when asked how you tell the difference between boys and girls, said: "Boys burp and run faster." A 4-year-old, similarly knowledgeable about genital differences, told his teacher that he had gone to a pet shop the day before with his father and had seen two girl cats and two boy cats. When the teacher asked him how he knew which was which, he said: "My Dad turned them over, and he read the print" (S. Minne, personal communication). Even seasoned clinicians are startled by how difficult it is for children to develop the conceptions of sex and gender that we adults take for granted. Not until age 6–7 do nearly all children understand that sexual categorization is based on anatomy.

Before these categorizations are well established, children often believe that they can grow up to have babies in their tummies and have a penis at the same time. The wish to be both sexes is not uncommon in 2–3-years-olds. One 3-year-old boy, while sitting in his mother's lap, touched her breast and said, "Mum, when I grow up, will I have muscles like this?" She said, "No, boys have penises, and girls have breasts." He looked at her intently and said, "Mum you're wrong, I'm going to have both" (S. Minne, personal communication). In general, in very young children penis envy is no more common in girls than the wish to have breasts and to give birth to a baby is in a boy (Linday, 1994). Many children experience some degree of loss when they realize the limits that their body imposes on their experience—that is, that boys do not become pregnant and girls do not have penises (Fast, 1984).

In the preschool years sex categorization is fluid, lacks constancy and stability, and is based on external appearance: a change in haircut and clothes typically means a change in sex categorization. Before these constancies are established, a child might be quite sure that he is a boy or a girl and confused about whether he will grow up to be a man or a woman. This fluidity leaves great room for dynamically informed wishes to take hold, sometimes with great tenacity. The integration of the child's understanding of gender categorization with experiences of sexual impulses is a very complex process and is, as yet, poorly understood. (For early efforts to understand developing sexuality, see Roiphe & Galenson, 1981.)

Once children are able to reliably label their own gender and that of their peers, there is increased gender segregation—that is, a proclivity for playing with same-sex peers, an increased interest in same-sex toys and a decreased interest in opposite-sex toys, and, for girls, a significant decrease in aggression (Fagot, 1993). By age 3–4 peer groups become powerful reinforcers of sex categorization. By age 5–6 cross-sex interests are increasingly less tolerated. Negative feedback from peers, particularly for boys with cross-gender interests, is increasingly common from peers.

The child's construction of his/her gender identity is a slow and piecemeal process that is deeply rooted in the child's attachment relationships and, as such, will reflect the history of those relationships and its conflicts, including intergenerational conflicts. Eve Sedgwyck has observed that some families are more "gendery" than others. In some families family mythology, family conceptualization, and family preoccupations, especially with issues of power and abuse, are saturated with gender content. Leslie Gibson (1998), working with Arietta Slade and with me, studied the Adult Attachment Interviews (AAIs) of non-clinical mothers who were given the AAIs (George,

Kaplan, & Main, 1985) in their third trimester of pregnancy. She found that mothers with AAIs that were densely filled with gender content had children whose play at age 28 months was highly gender-stereotypic, whether it be same-sex or other-sex gender preoccupations—that is, boys whose play was highly male-stereotypic or female-stereotypic had mothers who were very preoccupied with gender even before their child was born. She also found that women with insecure [preoccupied] as against secure AAI classifications had more rigid and elaborated preoccupations with gender.

Cross-gender interests occur in both typical development and when developmental processes are disrupted. At times, cross-gender behaviour is a brief passing phase, often in response to a passing stress, particularly in the 2–3-year-old child. At other times it is an indicator of gender flexibility. At still other times it is a signal of psychological suffering and can reflect the beginning of significant emotional difficulties, culminating in enduring disturbances. When a child's cross-gender preoccupations are intense, persistent, rigid, and pervasive, the condition is defined as a Childhood Gender Identity Disorder in the DSM–IV (American Psychiatric Association, 1992).

The onset of CGID typically occurs in late infancy and toddlerhood.

Diagnostic issues

Diagnostic criteria for CGID

At present in the DSM–IV, CGID is one of a number of syndromes classified according to the content of the symptom, without any consideration of aetiology.

The DSM–IV criteria for CGID are as follows:

A. A strong and persistent cross-gender identification (not merely a desire for any perceived cultural advantages of being the other sex).

In children, as manifested by at least *four* of the following:

1. repeatedly stated desire to be, or insistence that he or she is, the other sex
2. in boys, preference for cross-dressing or simulating female attire; in girls, insistence on wearing only stereotypical masculine clothing

3. strong and persistent preferences for cross-sex roles in make-believe play or persistent fantasies of being the other sex
4. intense desire to participate in the stereotypical games and pastimes of the other sex
5. strong preference for playmates of the other sex.

B. Persistent discomfort with one's sex or sense of inappropriateness in the role of that sex.

In children, manifested by any of the following:

1. In boys, assertion that his penis or testes are disgusting or will disappear or assertion that it would be better not to have a penis, or aversion towards rough-and-tumble play and rejection of male stereotypical toys, games, and activities;
2. In girls, rejection of urinating in a sitting position, assertion that she has or grows a penis, or assertion that she does not want to grow breasts or menstruate, or marked aversion towards normative feminine clothing.

C. Not concurrent with a physical intersex condition.

D. The disturbance causes clinically significant distress or impairment in social, occupational, or other important areas of functioning.

(The criteria for GID are currently being considered for revision: Coates, 2005.)

Epidemiology

No reliable estimate exists for the incidence of childhood GID in the general population. Clinical experience indicates that it is an extremely rare syndrome. Boys are referred for evaluation more often than girls, with a ratio of observed cases of approximately 6:1 (Zucker, 2004). We do not know whether this is the true prevalence of the disorder or whether it reflects greater social acceptability of cross-gender behaviour in girls. No data exists suggesting variation in the frequency of the disorder by ethnicity or socio-economic class.

The long-range social adaptation of children with GID has not yet been systematically studied. Clinical studies of adolescents with extreme cross-gender behaviour have found a high incidence of peer-relation difficulties, depression, and suicidal behaviour (Bradley, Zucker, Gladding, et al., 1984; Zucker & Bradley, 1995). In a study of suicidal behaviour in adults, Harry (1983) found that, among men, high levels of cross-gender behaviour in childhood were associated with suicidal behaviour in adulthood. This obtained whether the adults were homosexual or heterosexual.

There are far fewer studies of girls with childhood gender identity problems; thus, this report focuses primarily on boys with childhood GID.

Clinical presentation

CGID is a readily recognized syndrome characterized by persistent cross-gender fantasies and behaviour. The child intensely dislikes being a boy or a girl and actively wishes to be of the other gender. Although precursors of the disorder can sometimes be seen in a 1-year-old, the disorder usually first emerges between the ages of 2 and 3. Thus, the onset of the disorder occurs at a time when there is a major thrust in the development of an autonomous sense of self as separate from the mother, but before the establishment of a relatively stable sense of gender and of object constancy (Mahler, Pine, & Bergman, 1975).

The 2–3-year-old boy with GID will show a prolonged and marked preference for his mother's or sister's clothing and will lack the flexible interest seen in typical 2-year-olds who enjoy dressing up in everyone's clothes, Mummy's as well as Daddy's, sister's as well as brother's. The cross-gender fantasy will also incorporate the mother's activities, and the boy will engage in behaviours such as pretending to put on jewellery and make-up like Mummy, or he may insist on sitting to urinate. Moreover, his cross-gender interest will have an urgent and pressing quality to it that we usually associate with anxiety or even trauma in that it lacks the joy and easy spontaneity typical of children's play. In addition, boys with GID have a strong preference for playing with girls, usually alongside an avoidance of boy peers. They will prefer female stereotypical activities such as doll play, often with a special interest in Barbie, and will be interested in female stereotypic heroines such as Snow White and Cinderella (not heroes). By the time they are preschoolers, many boys with GID express anatomical dysphoria by voicing a wish to be rid of their penis, by attempting to hide it between their legs, or even in extreme cases by threatening to mutilate themselves.

In girls, the manifestations of GID are generally the mirror opposite of those that appear in boys—that is, the girl will prefer to imitate Daddy or big brother. She will be very rigid about wearing trousers on all occasions and, if required to wear a dress for a special occasion, may have an emotional meltdown that borders on a panic attack. She will insist that her hair be cut short and that she has a penis or will grow one when she gets older, and she will have a marked preference for the company and activities of boys alongside a marked avoidance of other girls, even those girls who share her interest in rough-and-tumble play.

It is important to note that it is common for young children without other clinical problems to have passing cross-gender fantasies and behaviour (Linday, 1994; Sandberg, Meyer-Bahlburg, Ehrhardt, & Yager, 1993). The issue is one of *degree* and the role that it is playing in the child's adaptive functioning. Once established, cross-gender symptoms evolve and develop as the child does. In untreated children, these symptoms sometimes remit and sometimes become progressively more autonomous from the forces that set them in motion and more and more deeply embedded in the child's defensive strategies and self-image.

Onset

Some cases appear to have a gradual onset. Others appear to have a very rapid onset, with the boy's cross-gender behaviour—including dressing up in Mummy's clothes, using her jewellery, her high-heeled shoes, and playing with her make-up—becoming consolidated in a period of days following some great stress and trauma in the family. Cross-gender behaviour in girls emerges at about the same time, between ages 2 and 3. Most cases, however, do not present for evaluation until the child is about 4 to 5. Often a teacher or paediatrician has told the parent either that this is a typical phase or that the child will grow out of it. Children who develop childhood GID overwhelmingly come from families where the symptom is family syntonic. Parents have usually found the child's behaviour amusing and cute and provide the child with endless Barbie dolls and pink tutus and so forth. These children are obviously not old enough to provide these for themselves, except in the cases where they make use of those objects belonging to a sister. One Dad said to me, "It's a pity he [his son] is not a girl, he looks so fabulous in a pink tutu." Parents of children with extreme gender issues usually "enjoy" their child's cross-gender behaviour until one day the child says that he hates being a boy and wants to be a girl or the girl says she hates being a girl and wants to be boy. Parents are usually deeply shaken when they realize that their child dislikes who he is and wants to be someone else. By age 5, boys with extreme cross-gender behaviour also begin to be excluded by their peers and are often mercilessly teased by other boys. This is the point where referrals are made to child clinicians.

Differential diagnosis

Prodromal phases of GID

A precocious 1½-year-old may already have a persistent fascination with his mother's clothes and with female heroines in books and videos and already be beginning to persistently imitate them in his play. Even at this very early age a careful diagnostic evaluation may uncover the child's use of cross-gender fantasies to manage anxiety.

The wish to be both genders

Prior to the age (roughly 2½ to 3½) when children learn to correctly label their own gender—that is: "I am a girl" or "I am a boy"—all children experience themselves as able to do and be all things male and female. Thus, little boys may believe that they can give birth, and little girls may believe that they may grow a penis while yet remaining girls. Once the child gives up this illusion, there is a loss involved. Some toddlers whose sense of self-worth is especially brittle or fragile may have trouble negotiating this period; they will show signs in their behaviour that they still harbour some of the old hopes of being both genders and express rage and envy at whichever parent or sibling seems to them to have dashed their hopes (see Fast, 1984, and Kubie, 1974, for further discussion). This is not GID: in GID the child wants to be *one* gender, the opposite one, not both, though if the child's distress at making this developmental transition is excessive, it is an indication of ongoing emotional strain in the child and may be an indication that the child and family need some help.

Gender flexibility

A different phenomenon involving cross-gender interests is sometimes observed in children who have a relatively well-established and positively affectively charged sense of their own gender identity. A little boy, for instance, may take up an interest in cooking, in growing flowers, or in play-acting both male and female roles, and may avoid rough-and-tumble play. A little girl may discover that she is a better athlete than most of the boys her age and begin to enjoy exercising her skills accordingly. These differences are the result of variations in character and temperament.

Transient cross-gender wishes and interests

Occasionally, one may see transitory reactions when children whose gender identity is reasonably well established show a sudden upsurge in cross-gender interests and behaviour in response to personal or familial crises. Although these behaviours may be intense, they rarely meet the full criteria for GID and they are short-lived, usually lasting less than three months.

Children with intersex conditions

In cases in which a true intersex condition exists—that is, where there is genital ambiguity—this condition may give rise to confusion about gender but rarely to GID (Meyer-Bahlburg, 1994). This is a different syndrome. However, an intersex child who is having significant confusion about his or her gender should receive help in sorting this out.

GID and later homosexual orientation

There are inconsistent data and significant controversy about the interpretation of existing research findings on the relationship between childhood GID and later sexual orientation. R. Green's early (1987b) longitudinal study of boys with GID found that, by adolescence, a sizable majority (75%) appeared to be developing a homosexual and/or bisexual orientation, while a substantial minority appeared to be developing a heterosexual orientation. Zucker and Bradley (1995) found the reverse with slightly younger children: the majority of boys with CGID appeared to be developing a heterosexual orientation. Green's study has been criticized as using a flawed methodology that resulted in an inflated estimate of homosexual outcome (Paul, 1993). A similar critique can be made of the Zucker and Bradley (1995) findings and Bailey and Zucker's (1995) findings. Green as well as Zucker and Bradley used Kinsey categories to assess heterosexual, bisexual, and homosexual outcomes in behaviour and fantasy, but they grouped the categories in a very particular way.

The Kinsey categories are the following:

0 exclusively heterosexual with no homosexual

1 predominantly heterosexual, only incidentally homosexual

2 predominantly heterosexual, but more than incidentally homosexual

3 equally heterosexual and homosexual

4 predominantly homosexual, but more than incidentally heterosexual

5 predominantly homosexual, only incidentally heterosexual

6 exclusively homosexual

Those considered heterosexual in the studies by Green (1987b), Zucker and Bradley (1995), and Bailey and Zucker (1995) were in Kinsey categories 0 and 1. All others were in a single category of 2 to 6. Thus bisexual and homosexual outcomes were lumped together, blurring real distinctions that may be there. One could conservatively conclude that a history of childhood GID may predispose boys to a have an increased likelihood, compared to the population at large, of developing a bisexual or homosexual outcome, but the frequency of this outcome is by no means a settled issue, and many children with GID become heterosexual. It is not uncommon in the analyses of adult heterosexual men to discover that as children they had gone through a phase of intense cross-gender interests, often occurring in the context of a maternal depression. Only a very small minority of adult homosexuals have a history of childhood GID, though many have a history of atypical gender interests that do not begin to reach the threshold of GID and do not involve a dislike of the self and a persistent wish to be of the other gender.

It is important to communicate to parents of children diagnosed with GID that not only are we unable at our current stage of knowledge to predict future sexual orientation in any individual child, but we are also unable, as yet, to understand the multiple complex factors that combine to determine later sexual orientation. Pathways to heterosexuality, bisexuality, and homosexuality appear to be very complex, involving multiple biological and experiential factors interacting at multiple levels of development to produce multiple pathways. Moreover there will probably be no linear relationships here, and main effects are likely to be in very complex interactions.

Multifactorial aetiology

Predisposing factors to GID are general, non-specific factors both in the child and in the parents that predispose the child to anxiety, such as unresolved trauma in the child's parents and the child having a sensitive reactive temperament and specific factors that predispose a child to use cross-gender fantasies as a solution to managing anxiety (Coates, 1990; Zucker & Bradley, 1995). Maternal and in some cases paternal selective attunement (Stern, 1985) to the child's cross-gender behaviour, which orient the child towards the specific "solution" of GID, can serve as powerful reinforcers of cross-gender behaviour. These children are trying to do what is expected of them. The cross-gender behaviour increases the child's sense of security because it pleases the parents and helps to keep the parents' own unresolved traumatic issues in check, albeit at great cost to the child in terms of emotional autonomy and authenticity. A comprehensive, fully integrated etiological model adequate to the description of all cases has yet to be achieved. In a majority of families, cascading anxiety, depression, and trauma will intersect with the child's temperament during a sensitive developmental period. There are multiple pathways to childhood GID, and not all of them have yet been descriptively detailed in the literature.

Temperamental factors

Despite extensive investigation, no direct evidence has been found to date that either genetic or hormonal influences are at work in the disorder. Indirect evidence from animal research and from spontaneously occurring endocrine disorders suggests that genes and hormones affect aspects of stereotypical gender-role behaviour such as rough-and-tumble play but does not directly affect gender identity (Ehrhardt & Meyer-Bahlburg, 1981).

General factors that would predispose children to a wide variety of disorders involve the indirect contribution of hormonal and genetic factors, the mode of operation of which in humans is still largely unknown, but which can be conceptualized in terms of temperament or constitutional differences in affect regulation (Bradley, 1985, 1990).

Boys with GID are less physically active than other boys; they avoid rough-and-tumble play with their peers and appear to be a subgroup of Kagan's (1989) shy, inhibited, slow-to-warm-up children who are anxious in the face of novelty (Coates, Hahn-Burke, & Wolfe, 1994). They may also have difficulty managing aggression and expressing it in socially acceptable ways. We have growing evidence that the predisposition to this temperament is genetic but expression of this behaviour is also highly influenced by experience, as the work of Steve Suomi has taught us (Suomi, 1991).

One would expect that boys so endowed would show greater-than-average need for an attachment relationship—and, indeed, this is what one sees clinically. Such children are often highly reliant upon caregivers to provide them with clues as to whether a situation is safe and to help them to regulate their anxiety. Though anxious in new situations and slow to warm up, boys often eventually make intense attachments in which they then do not appear to be shy. They are highly attuned to others' affective experience and readily pick up the slightest emotional cues.

Beyond the need for and readiness to engage in an attachment bond, these boys also seem to have special sensory sensitivities (Coates, Hahn-Burke, Wolfe, Shindledecker, & Nierenberger, 1994; Coates & Wolfe, 1995; Stoller, 1968). They are unusually reactive to odours and colour and are often responsive to sound and texture. Not only do these boys appear more alive to the sensory world, but they are more vulnerable to it.

Far less is known about the constitutional predisposition to GID in girls. Clinical reports indicate that girls are the mirror opposite of boys in terms of rough-and-tumble play and activity level. They appear on the surface to be bold and are highly invested in athletic activities, and research also suggests that they have high activity levels and exhibit high levels of both externalizing and internalizing behavioural symptoms (Zucker & Bradley, 1995). Despite their apparent extroversion, however, our clinical impression is that girls have as high an anxiety level as boys predisposed to cross-gender identifications, but because of their temperament they often manage their anxiety with oppositional and counterphobic defensive strategies.

Associated psychopathology in boys

Most prominent among the associated features of GID is separation anxiety (Coates & Person, 1985; Zucker, Bradley, & Lowry Sullivan, 1996). Approximately two thirds of boys with GID also meet the criteria for a DSM–III–R separation anxiety disorder, and most of the remaining third have significant symptoms of separation anxiety (Coates & Person, 1985; Zucker, Bradley, & Lowry Sullivan, 1996). Three quarters of children with GID are insecurely attached (Birkenfeld-Adams, Zucker and Bradley, 1998). Boys with GID also tend to have fears of bodily injury and symptoms of depression.

Boys with GID have an overall degree of psychopathology that is similar to other psychiatrically referred children as defined by the CBCL (Zucker & Bradley, 1995). Although few systematic studies of psychological functioning in girls have been published, Zucker and Bradley (1995), using the CBCL, found comparable levels of psychopathology in girls with GID as in boys

Parental psychopathology

Maternal depression, anxiety, and unresolved trauma

The parents of children with GID have ongoing problems in affect regulation (Bradley, 2000). In mothers this often presents as maternal depression or anxiety (Marantz & Coates, 1991) and in fathers as anxiety, depression, and/or substance abuse (Wolfe, 1990), often accompanied by explosive behaviour.

GID most often arises in the context of the loss of the emotional availability of the mother, usually due to depression, anxiety, or a traumatic experience. Chronically anxious and depressed states in the mother are well known, in and of themselves, to have deep and far-reaching impact on the child's development (Emde, 1980; 1983). The abrupt loss of the primary care-taker to her own depression may be likened psychologically to a confrontation with what André Green (1986) describes as the "dead mother"—a mother who is present but not there and who is therefore gone but cannot be mourned. The child of a depressed mother loses not only the mother's emotional availability to help him regulate his anxiety, but also her mirroring and reflective capacities that allow a child to know his own mind. In a young child such a loss is catastrophic and threatens to destabilize not only the child's ability to regulate negative affect but also the child's developing sense of self. The child will search for any means within his capacity to restore this emotional connection.

In an early study of 25 mothers, nearly 70% described events that they experienced as traumatic around the time of the birth of their son or within the first two years of their son's life—Coates, unpublished data). Recent in-depth pilot studies using the Adult Attachment Interview (George, Kaplan, & Main, 1985) to assess parental attachment status found that in the first five families studied, mothers and fathers of boys diagnosed with GID exhibited an insecure state of mind with regard to their own past attachment relationships—that is, these parents *as adults* exhibit internal working models of attachment relationships that reflect insecure attachment histories (Cook, 1999; Hahn-Burke, 1998). All five of the mothers were classified as preoccupied and unresolved in relation to trauma. Of six fathers, five were classified as preoccupied, one as secure, and all six as unresolved in respect to trauma. Peter Fonagy reported to me that none of the 100 clinic-referred children in their studies at the Anna Freud Centre had two parents that were unresolved in respect to mourning and loss, which brings into relief how extreme the traumatic issues are for families of boys with GID. Importantly, many parents also had experienced attachment-related unresolved traumas and losses from their own past histories that had become organized in their memory around gender content. These unresolved traumas left them vulnerable, when such experiences were re-activated in their current parenting experiences, to displaying the frightened and frightening behaviour (Main & Hesse, 1990) that has been linked to disorganized attachments with the child and to being highly reactive to the child's gender-coded behaviour.

Clinical experience is compatible with these research findings. Very often, over the course of treatment if not in the initial evaluation, it becomes clear that the mother's depression was precipitated by traumatic events within the family—events that engender massive anxiety and clinically significant depression, often accompanied by rageful outbursts in the mother, rendering her suddenly and emotionally inaccessible and frightening to her son (Coates, Friedman, & Wolfe, 1991; Coates & Moore, 1997) and leading to the derailment of the mother–son attachment bond. In many cases the consolidation of the cross-gender behaviour occurs in the wake of the traumatic loss of the mother's accessibility, and it, in turn, is often partially successful in restoring the derailed relationship to the mother.

The effect of the trauma on the mother is almost invariably compounded by the father's inability, due to his own limitations or psychopathology, to intervene effectively in helping his wife to cope by taking over her function as the primary caretaker. The father may withdraw, making himself unavailable to his wife and son. In addition, paternal psychopathology may present in forms of substance abuse and hyperaggressive behaviour that lead the sensitive boy to want to disidentify with the father (Cook, 1999). The role of unresolved trauma in parents of girls with GID has not yet been studied, though there are a number of clinical reports of rapid onset of GID after a specific trauma.

Psychodynamics in boys with GID

Though it is impossible to get a perfectly clear window on the mind of a 2- or a 3-year-old, what seems to happen in many cases is that boys attempt to manage their separation anxiety, triggered by the mother's emotional inaccessibility, with a fantasy solution in which they imagine themselves as "being Mummy" rather than "being with Mummy". In effect, they substitute an alien introject (see Fonagy, Gergely, Jurist, & Target, 2002) for a metabolized identification and an object relationship. Imitation of a lost or emotionally absent person is a familiar psychological mechanism, and at this young developmental age, Minna Emch (1944) argues, imitation is used by the child when he or she cannot make sense of the mother's behaviour as a means of attempting to understand the behaviour. I believe that imitating Mummy's physical appearance or gestures becomes a substitute for having access to her mind and in turn to one's self as Fonagy's work has so clearly demonstrated (Fonagy et al., 2002). Importantly, it is not only the mother that is lost in this solution but the authentic self as well (Abraham & Torok, 1984).

Other boys may manage parental inaccessibility by becoming hypervigilant to the parents' selective attunement to their passing cross-gender behaviour. The cross-gender behaviour comes to serve multiple functions, both intrapsychic and interpersonal. In situations in which the mother has become depressed, the child may altruistically sacrifice his authentic development by transforming himself into an "other" that he imagines will help to restore his mother. When the boy's cross-gender behaviour succeeds at least momentarily in engaging and enlivening the "dead mother"—she may find it cute or funny—the boy may experience, in his mother's enlivened response, a partial and temporary restoration of the lost mother–child emotional relationship (Coates & Wolfe, 1995). In this psychological scenario, the mother's selective attunement to the child's cross-gender behaviour would serve as a particularly powerful external reinforcer of the cross-gender behaviour in the boy.

The child's cross-gender fantasies generally interlock with the parents' internal worlds in various and precise ways. But though the specific intersection of the child's dynamics with the parental dynamics in this disorder can take a myriad of forms and there is no set relation between the two, certain presentations are frequently observed. For example, by becoming a girl, a boy may be offering himself to his mother as a replacement for a lost female child or other deceased relative, the loss of whom has not been adequately mourned. Often the boy is reassuring the mother, and sometimes the father, that he will not become a stereotypic male who, they unconsciously fear, may trigger memories of psychological or physical abuse that could, in turn, bring on their own intense aggression towards the child. In this way the child protects the parents from their potential for affect dysregulation in relation to him.

Clinical experience has repeatedly shown that the child's cross-gender fantasy most often constitutes a "solution" that works for the mother, the child, and often the father as well. Along similar lines, a father may be unconsciously gratified by his son's symptoms if he experiences the cross-gender behaviours as satisfying an intense—but denied—need for nurturance from the father's own longed-for but emotionally inaccessible mother. Fearing that becoming male means turning into an aggressive monster—a belief that has come about through his experience in his particular family—the boy may also disidentify from a father whom he perceives as insensitive or as abusive and destructive to his mother (Cook, 1999). Though there are infinite numbers of ways in which parental dynamics may intersect with the child's dynamic solution, the child's symptoms will inevitably have powerful meaning for both parents, and the exploration of this meaning will be critical in helping the family to find alternative methods for regulating dysphoric affect.

Once the cross-gender fantasy is established and successfully reduces traumatic levels of anxiety, it becomes readily available for use in less traumatic situations in which the child has not yet developed effective coping strategies, including brief periods of maternal loss (such as short business trips) and brief episodes of maternal emotional unavailability, separations, and transitions, and occasions that evoke anxiety about the child's aggression. Once the child invents his "solution", the increasing autonomy that it gives him from his family also serves to perpetuate the defence. Family dynamics and the additional complication of increasing social ostracism by male peers (preventing typical peer socialization of gender) will also all interact and further lock in this solution.

For children with GID, no matter how creative and reparative a solution the cross-gender fantasy may be, the rigidity and pervasiveness of the preoccupation is costly intrapsychically and interpersonally. The child's psychic energy is taken up by the needs of others, leaving little room for autonomy and authenticity. In some extreme cases, the resulting dysphoria may be manifest in preoccupations with suicide and, in rare instances, attempts to mutilate one's own genitalia. In all cases, a child's sense of authenticity is compromised. The boy's suffering can sometimes be obscured by a manic-like presentation that can initially be confusing to the clinician. For example, one little boy, who during his evaluation drew a very elaborate and colourful picture of a lady that included a brightly coloured rainbow, was asked, after he had been in therapy and continued to draw similar pictures, what was at the end of his rainbow. He responded, "A big black pit filled with dead bodies and bones." On the cover of

Zucker and Bradley's 1995 book on childhood GID you see a brightly coloured picture of a girl skipping in the sunshine and beside her a tombstone with her own initials on it. It is not uncommon for boys with GID to use manic defences to cover dysphoric affect. These manic drawings are similar to the "over-bright" drawings of children whose attachment style is disorganized or dissociated.

In some children a sense of loneliness and intense psychological suffering is expressed directly. They may volunteer that "nobody likes me" or "I wish I was dead" or "why did God make me a boy?" As treatment proceeds, and some of their creativity is freed up, these children are often capable of producing remarkably moving and detailed accounts of their suffering. One boy, "Colin", in a vignette I illustrate later, marshalled his artistic talents to produce a series of drawings entitled "My Story", in which with *Guernica*-like figures he portrayed the terror and psychological pain of being transformed into a woman against his will. Another boy told a story in which a boy is informed by a monster that the only way to make contact with what he described as his "dead" mother was to turn into her.

Psychodynamics in girls with GID

In girls, the constellation of dynamic factors appears to be different, as does the intersection with temperament. When a girl with a sensitive, inhibited temperament is traumatized by sudden maternal withdrawal, clinical experience suggests that she will respond not with cross-gender fantasies, but with the development of a separation anxiety disorder or an exaggerated hyperfemininity. Both rigid hyperfemininity in girls and rigid hypermasculinity in boys are also disorders of gender, but they often present as overanxious disorders or, later in childhood, as eating disorders in girls or as conduct disorders in boys.

Systematic research on girls with GID is only just beginning, but clinical experience suggests that in addition to a bold temperament, predisposing family factors in one pathway to the disorder are the combination of a hyperaggressive father and one who devalues women in combination with a mother who is perceived as ineffective or who devalues women herself. The girl may identify with the father as a means of disidentifying with a devalued mother or with the father perceived as the aggressor in an effort to protect the mother and herself: "I will become strong and valued like Daddy, so that I can protect Mummy who is fragile and vulnerable, and myself as well." Girls with GID often experience the father as psychologically or physically abusive (Zucker & Bradley, 1995). In these cases, identification with the aggressor is an important aspect of the defensive solution that helps the girl to feel safer. Another less common pathway involves girls who begin to have fantasies of being boys after their mother has experienced a life-threatening gynaecological problem. These girls develop the belief that remaining a girl exposes them to the threat of annihilation.

In either pathway, girls are usually also responding to powerful issues in the family constellation, such as a mother or father idealizing males and simultaneously devaluing females.

The extremely low incidence of GID in girls as compared to boys indicates that a multiplicity of risk factors must be simultaneously present and operate with a rare intensity to produce the disorder. To be borne constantly in mind in attempting to understand the disorder in both boys and girls is that no matter how readily GID may fit in with prevailing family dynamics and interpersonal realities, it still represents an intrapsychic solution to the management of anxiety about annihilation, separation, and aggression in the child. The cost to the child of the defensive strategies for managing such severe anxieties through cross-gender symptoms is continuing to develop a false and inauthentic self, a self based primarily upon the needs of others (Winnicott, 1954), impairing the capacity to feel real and to feel recognized, known, and nurtured by others.

Case vignettes

The following case is a modification of one provided in the chapter on childhood GID in the *DC: 0–3 Casebook* (Coates & Wolfe, 1997; for a full account see Coates & Moore, 1997).

The case of Colin

> Colin was referred at the age of 3½ to a mental health practitioner by his nursery school teacher because of his inability to get along with other children. If he did not get his way, he would hit

them, or else he would scowl, cross his arms, and turn his face to the wall. Moreover, from the perspective of the nursery school, his current behaviour represented a marked change from the time that he had been evaluated for entrance into the nursery programme nearly eight months earlier. A consultation revealed that he also had extensive preoccupations with cross-gender fantasies that included a belief that he was going to grow up to be a girl. He openly stated that he wished to be a girl and that he hated being a boy. He believed he was born a girl and that if you wore girls' clothes, you could really become a girl and "not just for pretend." Since the age of 2½ he had regularly dressed in his mother's clothes and would spend long periods of time cross-dressing while observing himself intently in front of a mirror. He was intensely interested in jewellery and make-up, he repetitively stroked the hair of Barbie dolls, and he had a marked interest in heroines (and avoided heroes) in fairy tales such as Snow White and Rumpelstiltskin. He also showed a notable lack of interest in playing with other boys.

When Colin first came to our centre, he needed his mother to stay with him throughout the first interviews. He was initially physically clingy, preoccupied with his mother's well-being and very attentive to her affect. He was overtly solicitous, asking for example: "Mummy, are you okay?" His attentiveness to her—"That's a pretty dress, Mummy" and "Mummy, I love you"—and her response to that attentiveness was reversed in terms of the ordinary roles of child and parent—similar to children with disorganized attachments—in that he functioned as her protector rather than the reverse.

Despite his initial inhibition, Colin was readily engaged by the examiners. He was hypervigilant to the adults, particularly their facial expressions and what they were wearing. He had no interest in toys or in playing, and his initial presentation was that of a precocious, compliant, overly attuned adult who responded to meeting with two new adults in a singularly unchildlike way.

He said, "I hate myself, I don't want to be me. I want to be someone else. I want to be a girl." He felt that it was better to be a girl because you "could wear pretty clothes" and because "boys were too rough".

Family background, development, and context for the onset of symptoms

Mrs S remembers her pregnancy and the first year of Colin's life as uneventful. She recalls Colin at age 1 as a "laughing baby" with an easy-going temperament who was loving, gentle, and "always happy".

For both parents, the category of gender was highly salient in their own lives and in their perceptions of their growing son. For the father, Colin's gentle temperament brought to mind his own troubled boyhood where his sensitivity and timidity had left him ill-equipped to deal with an angry, inaccessible, and explosive alcoholic mother or to relate to either his father or brother, both bold, aggressive types. His principal concern was that Colin should develop a sense of his own "power"—he found Colin's cross-gender interests "interesting" and seemed selectively attuned to this aspect of his behaviour.

When Colin's mother was 3 years old, her sickly brother was born, and her mother virtually abandoned her care to the father. The family became split along the lines of mother and son forming one unit and father and daughter another, at least until the mother reached adolescence. Furthermore, in the mother's family of origin, boys were enormously overvalued compared to girls. Her younger brother had many "male privileges" that were very distressing to her. For example, only he was allowed to have second helpings on food; she could only have a second helping if any remained after the brother had taken all that he wanted. Having a son was thus potentially problematic for her, since feelings of loss and deprivation were linked in her own childhood to male privilege and the loss of her mother's emotional availability.

Shortly after Colin's second birthday, his family planned a five-day trip abroad, but Colin became ill before their departure. Colin and his mother stayed behind, and his father and his grandmother left for Europe for a week. His mother reported that during their absence Colin became inconsolable: "He cried until his father and grandmother returned." Both parents agree that Colin's behaviour changed at this point in time. He became anxious and was now markedly clingy and extremely sensitive to all separations.

Mrs S, concerned that Colin "did not have enough companionship", decided to have a second child. She was also eager to repeat her earlier pleasurable experiences with Colin as an infant. However, this time her pregnancy ended in tragedy: amniocentesis led to the foetal diagnosis of Down's syndrome. In addition to doubting the wisdom of carrying such a pregnancy to term, both parents questioned their capacity to raise a severely disabled child, should the infant survive. They were also deeply concerned about the impact such an experience would have on Colin. Given these considerations, they chose to terminate the pregnancy.

The amniocentesis had also revealed that the foetus was a female, and during the three-week waiting period prior to the abortion Mrs S developed elaborate fantasies about this girl child. She named the foetus "Miriam" after a revered teacher and felt grateful for the waiting period prior to the abortion as this allowed her "to get to know Miriam". She withdrew from Colin and became preoccupied with Miriam. She had fantasies of sewing dresses for Miriam and of giving her to her mother so that she would "have something to live for". After the abortion, though her husband experienced a pronounced grief reaction, Mrs S did not. Though she felt chronically depressed and anxious thereafter, Mrs S did not connect these feelings with the loss of the baby.

Colin's cross-gender behaviour began within weeks of the abortion, and it rapidly assumed the driven quality characteristic of children with the full syndrome of CGID. Colin began to insist that he dress up in his mother's clothes. He began to pretend that he was a girl. Mrs S seemed very attuned to his new preoccupation and took numerous pictures of him cross-dressed. Colin seemed to have sensed his mother's preoccupation with a girl, and in his imitation of girls we believe he attempted to repair his mother's depression by replacing the lost girl and thereby restoring the derailed attachment that occurred during her pregnancy and the aftermath of the abortion.

After two years of therapy, when his cross-gender behaviour was no longer repetitively enacted, he showed a marked increase in his capacity to represent his experience symbolically, both verbally and nonverbally. During this time one evening at home he drew a series of drawings that he called "Colin's Story". He asked his mother to write down a caption that he dictated for each of the nine pictures. The result was a pictorial and verbal narrative of his sense of being colonized by his mother's needs (Coates, Friedman, & Wolfe, 1991; for a detailed description of this case, see Coates & Moore, 1997.)

Colin's Story

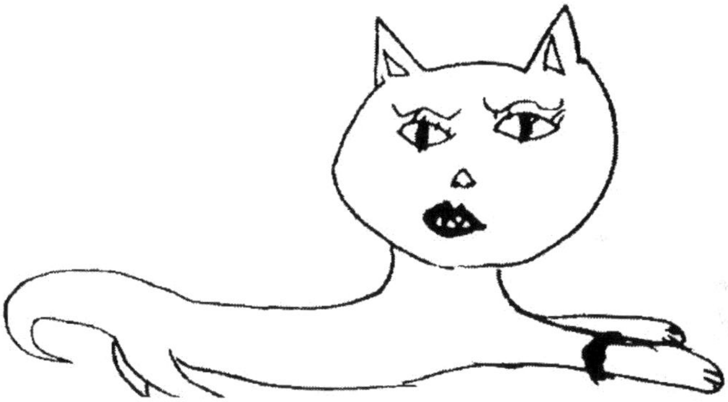

The cat is angry that she's turning into a lady.
She doesn't know why she's turning into a lady.

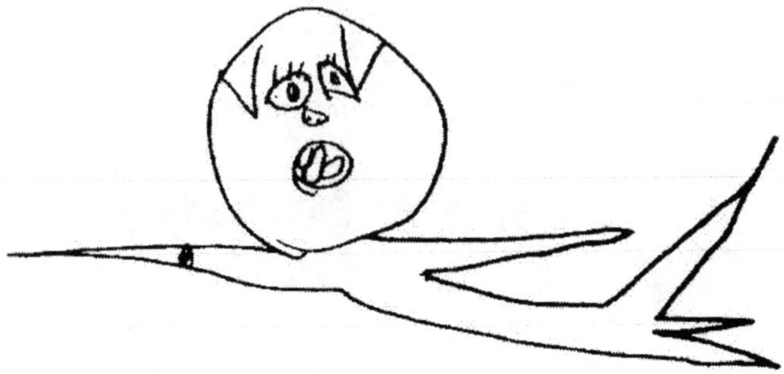

She's screaming because she's so mad
she's turning into a lady.

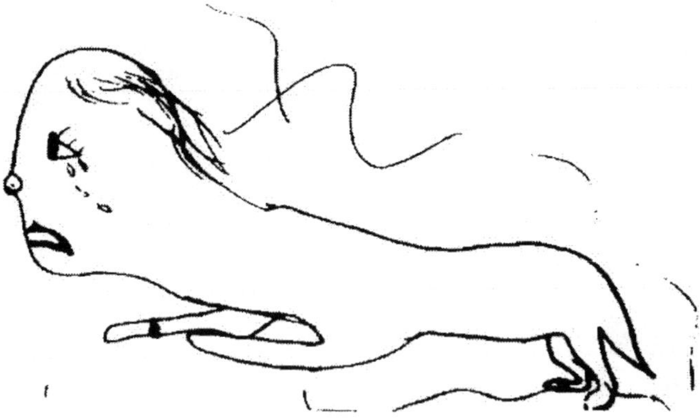

She's crying and sad she's turning into a lady.
She already has hair.

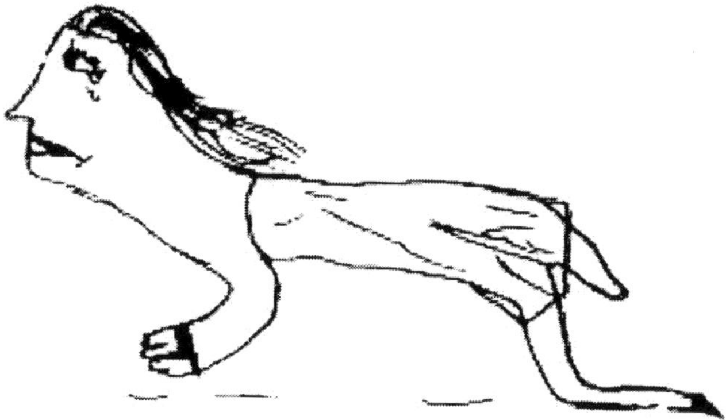

She's crying and she's almost a lady.
She still has her tail.

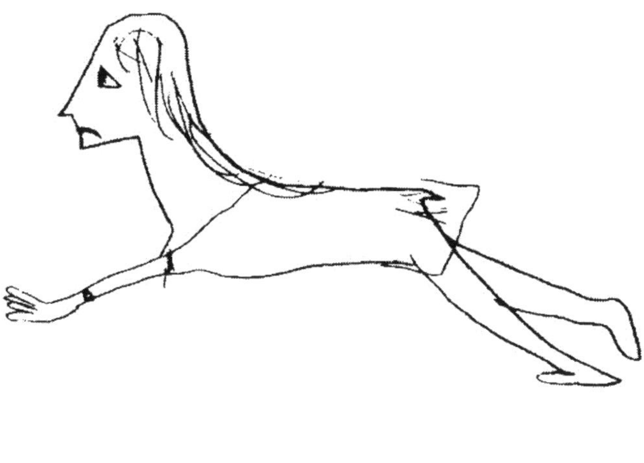

She almost lost her tail.

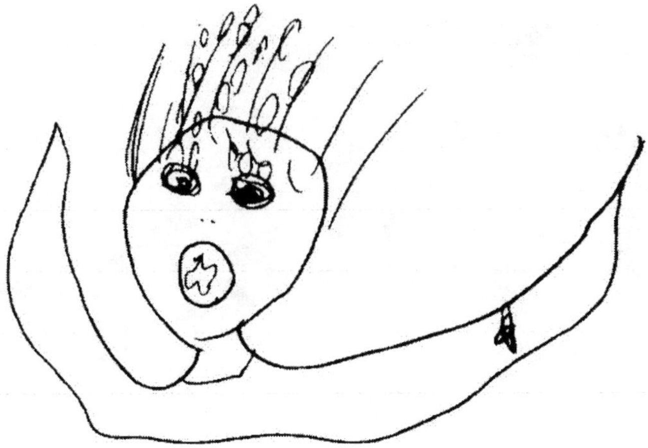

She's screaming so loudly her hair is going up
and her tears are going up.

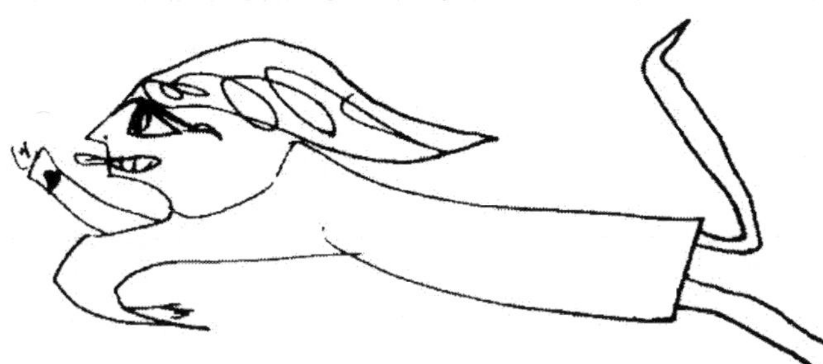

She's so mad she bit her tongue and lost her tears.

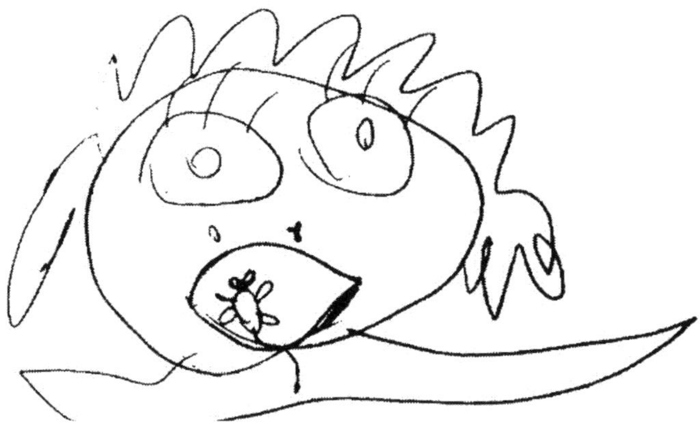

She's eating her mother and she looks like a weirdo.
She's mad but not at her mother.
She ate her mother because she's so mad.

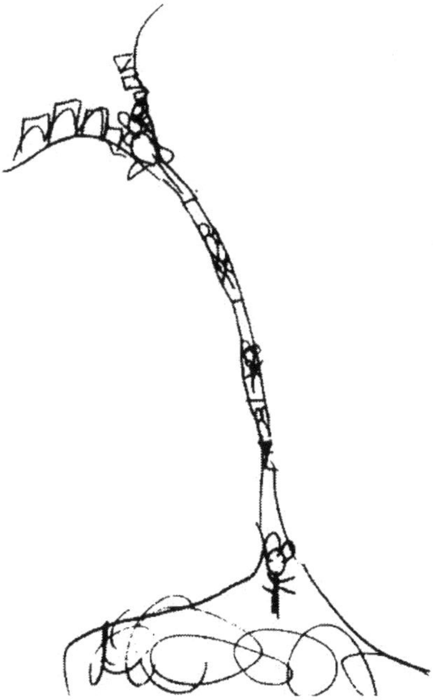

She's going to the bathroom;
she got her mother out
and her mother is dead.
She's not sad.

The story depicts an experience of being taken over from the outside, resulting in a sense of annihilation of the self as Colin is transformed against his will into another. This experience, first represented in terms of annihilation, becomes fused in the later pictures with imagery expressive of age-appropriate castration anxiety. His profound anguish and pain is poignantly expressed. His rage is depicted in the primitive incorporative imagery of eating his mother. When he attempts to put this primitive rage into words, there is a breakdown in his cognitive coherence. What is most striking is that the representation and fantasy of the physical incorporation of the mother leads both to a fusion with her and a destruction of her as a separate individual while simultaneously leading to the elimination of the affective experience of being sad and, presumably, mad. Colin, as most children, has altruistically sacrificed his own autonomy and authenticity in an attempt to shore up his mother's depression and to protect both his mother and his father from unresolved issues of trauma from their own upbringing.

Children with GID need to be in intensive psychoanalytic psychotherapy where the parents are simultaneously in a coordinated treatment with the child's treatment. Work with children should be aimed at helping them to resolve their separation anxiety and to develop effective coping strategies for managing anxiety, particularly around issues of separation and aggression. They need help in developing a mind of their own, where they can experience a genuine sense of authenticity. Work with parents needs to focus on resolving issues of unresolved trauma to help free the child from intergenerational transfer of trauma and should also be aimed at helping parents to become able to respond to their child's needs and temperament in both sensitive and an age-appropriate ways. When these underlying issues are addressed, rigid cross-gender symptoms become resolved without having to address the cross-gender symptoms directly with the child.

SUMMARY

For a gender identity disorder to consolidate in late infancy and early toddlerhood, multiple factors must interact in a sensitive time period before the child has developed a relatively consolidated sense of his or her own gender. Both non-specific factors, such as unresolved trauma in the parents and a predisposition to anxiety in the child, and specific factors involving parental selective attunement to cross-gender behaviour and preoccupations in the child must come together during a sensitive developmental time period.

An interlocking of the child's dynamics with the family dynamics is necessary to bring about the disorder. The parents' selective attunement to the child's cross-gender behaviour serves as a powerful reinforcer of cross-gender behaviour that may otherwise just be a passing phase. In both girls and boys, the rigid, persistent and pervasive cross-gender symptoms of GID enable the child to achieve a partial success in that they help the child to feel more secure in relation to the parents, to restore, in fantasy if not in real life, his or her attachment security, and to stabilize both parents' difficulties with affect regulation. The partial success of this defensive strategy in stabilizing family systemic issues around unresolved trauma is a powerful motivating force that quickly becomes self-perpetuating, but it comes at great cost to the child, who develops an alien self, as the important work of Fonagy and Target has taught us: it is a self deprived of internal flexibility, a sense of autonomy, and authenticity.

Commentary

Sheila Spensley

It is important and timely to be reconsidering the subject of gender identity and sexuality. While Western societies become increasingly concerned with questions of sexuality, fears in relation to disturbances of sexuality (including the abuse of children) are, paradoxically, debated within a contemporary culture in which a general debasement of mature adult sexuality proliferates. There are trends towards treating sexuality as if it were a speciality relationship technique to be treated separately from affectional and attachment ties and, indeed, accorded greater value. In contrast, Freud's libido theory ("The libido theory and narcissism", Lecture XXVI in 1916–17) of sexuality had at its heart a strong argument for enlarging the concept of sexuality to recognize its central significance for all human achievement. He advanced the idea that sexuality imbued all the instinctual drives, supporting this view with the presumption of the existence of a special chemical factor linking the sex glands and the central nervous system. His theory was based on the scientific knowledge available at the time, but it was an idea that actually anticipated the discovery of the sex hormones.

At a stroke, as it were, he had produced a theory of sexuality that accounted for the sexual aberrations, the neurotic and the psychotic disorders. Freud envisaged the infant as coming into the world trailing "germs of sexuality" that imbue all of the other impulses and instinctual drives that serve self-preservation. This endows the infant with maximal potential for a full libidinal thrust towards life, as well as the potential for the whole gamut of aberrations or perversions from that primary aim, which are manifested in neurotic and psychotic disorders. His emphasis on the central part played by sexuality in the neuroses was matched by his insistence (as early as 1896) on the significance of the early childhood years in the origins of certain phenomena connected with sexual life and "the part played in sexuality by the infantile factor". In this he included the polymorphous opportunities for sexualized gratification via all other organs of the body, which he regarded as a fundamental human characteristic.

Freud ended his *Three Essays on the Theory of Sexuality* (1905d) with the cautionary note that further knowledge of biology was needed to substantiate a libido theory of the personality that claimed such a critical role for the sexual instinctual impulses. He would, no doubt, be gratified by today's advances in empirical knowledge and understanding, which offer further support for his hypotheses. Susan Coates's chapter presents research-derived knowledge of child development alongside her clinical observation, and it is particularly welcome to child psychotherapists to have these two fields brought into conjunction, to augment the work of each.

Gender identity disorder

Coates begins with a helpful chronology in relation to infants' capacities to experience and identify themselves and others. The amusing anomalies that she describes in relation to the gap between a child's intellectual and emotional knowledge of sexual differences—the capacity to spot the difference between the sexes at 6 months, which by the age of 2 years requires extra clues—seems to endorse Freud's (1915c) view of an early unconscious awareness of libidinal forces that suffuses the infant from birth. However, the disparity will also be of particular note to those clinicians with an interest in the concepts employed by Wilfred Bion, whose evolutionary theory of thinking begins with *preconceptions* as the building blocks of the capacity to think. That is to say, the infant is biologically wired with certain preconceptions that provide a kind of unconscious blueprint for sexuality and reproduction. The evidence Coates presents for a slow and erratic construction of gender identity reiterates the formative influences of early experience and the history of attachment relationships.

The diagnostic categorizations of GID are in agreement about the significant degree of distress and suffering that is caused in addition to the presenting symptoms of the condition, which has its onset around the point of separation experience and autonomous functioning at age 2–3 years. That the level of anxiety is severe is underscored by associated depression and suicide in adolescence and mental anguish; this was a factor in the case to which I refer below. Alongside this is the clinical evidence that disorders of affect are pervasive in the families of children with GID. Significantly, the incidence of GID among cases of true intersex genital ambiguity is rare and is, I think, a sharp reminder that dysphoria concerning the genitalia arises in the mind, not the body, of the sufferer, although it is not perceived that way by the child or the adolescent. A further characteristic of some interest is that the condition is six times more likely to occur in boys than in girls, and this difference may provide an avenue for the further exploration of the disorder.

In Coates's lucid account of the clinical presentation and the childhood family experience of children with GID, one feature emerges again and again, from exhaustive investigations of all the possible factors contributing to the syndrome: the presence of extreme anxiety, which she sees as the key to the psychodynamics of the condition. Affect regulation is a pervasive problem within families who have a child with GID, and she sees the condition as a strategy for managing high anxiety. She also draws attention to the complex multiplicity of factors that interact during a sensitive period for the consolidation of identity in the child. Severe anxiety in the child may be met by parents who themselves carry a legacy of anxiety that conflates the problem of management. As a strategy for managing anxiety, GID appears to provide some defence and a semblance of family equilibrium against overwhelming threat, but it does so at enormous cost to the child.

My own experience of this syndrome is limited, but it does confirm Coates's formulation of the psychodynamics as a defence against separation anxiety and one that involves a sense of "being the mother, rather than *being with* a mother". Clinically, this is a defence commonly encountered in children with psychotic and borderline conditions and has grave implications for personal and cognitive development. Such children cannot achieve identity *with* the object because they retreat into being identical *to* the object. A real subject–object world of relationships is obliterated along with experience of separateness and "twoness". As Coates points out, the primary symptomatology concerns internalizing, not externalizing, as defined by the CBCL.

Coates describes GID as "an intrapsychic solution to the management of very severe anxiety "which results in a false, inauthentic sense of self". This I fully agree with, but I want to consider a further possibility: that it extends to a deeper level, to a delusional sense of self. In GID, the "internal working model" of relationship is not reality-based, but fantasy-based. Identity of the self is generated not through recognition of the object and the model of dependency on another human being, but by an urgent drive to find refuge *from* dependency, which seems to constitute an existential threat of overwhelming anxiety. Winnicott (1956), Ogden (1989), and Tustin (1981) describe this catastrophic state of terror, respectively, as a dread of "failure to go on being", "organismic anxiety", and "the fate worse than death". The terror and panic involved is to be distinguished from separation anxiety in that this is not about loss of the object, but about loss of the sense of existence—hence the flight from reality to fantasy to preserve some illusion of selfhood. In the case of psychotic children, we know that the therapeutic task involved in restoring a sense of reality is a formidable one, so I am most interested to learn whether there is, as yet, evidence to suggest that the differences of degree in relation to GID may allow for more hopefulness in relation to treatment outcome.

In GID, loss of the emotional availability of the mother has been identified as a prime factor, and this is considered in the context of maternal anxiety or depression. In the latter case the mother may be present but "not there" in her capacity for reflection or as a container of anxiety. Adult Attachment Interviews have demonstrated that the majority of parents of boys diagnosed with GID have insecure AAI classifications and, furthermore, that they are also more likely to have had unresolved experiences involving loss or trauma. Unresolved and insecure internal models of attachment in parents do not favour the development of parenting skills with optimal capacities for emotional containment.

I would now like to turn to the case vignette to consider the clinical material from the perspective of emotional containment as a prerequisite of secure identity.

Case material

Colin is referred by his nursery school because of his uncontainment; he wants the world to conform to his wishes and cannot brook frustration. It is also clear that the family history of his parents is one characterized by inadequate emotional containment, which is likely to compromise their parenting capacities. Colin's father had had the experience of an explosive, alcoholic mother and an aggressive father. His mother had felt abandoned by her own mother in favour of an ailing brother. Colin's attachment bond with his mother seems to have been problematic from an early age since, at the age of 2, it was separation from his father that precipitated his symptoms and mother's presence does not seem to have been enough to compensate for the loss of father. Colin's mother then drops him, at the age of 3, in her preoccupation with fantasies about her pre-abortion baby, misdirecting her attention from her real live baby Colin.

Given this state of affairs, I want to consider the catastrophe of GID not only in terms of loss of emotional containment but in relation to the loss of the underlying preconception of a link with an object that is either not confirmed by the infant's experience or is broken by adverse experience. Bion's (1962) concept of containment represents a link, a tensile link, between a container and that which it contains, and the prototype for emotional linking is the fundamental biological link intrinsic to the activities of feeding and sexuality—that is, the mouth–nipple and penis–vagina model. In Bion's theory, this primary model, which sustains physical life, transmutes to provide the same model for generating psychic life. The theory is consistent with Freud's view of the universal nature of unconscious sexuality, so that it is less than surprising to find that disruptions in the experience of emotional containment should result in disturbances not only of interpersonal relationships, but also of intrapersonal experience of the self and of identity, as the case material shows. "In all cases, a child's sense of authenticity is compromised" (Coates).

Indeed, the sexual link as a fundamental concept in thinking is universal and embedded in the language. Throughout the building industry, tradesmen, craftsmen, and technicians rely on the concept of male and female in relation to the components of construction. There is a line in Alan Bennett's play *Forty Years On* (1968), where a sardonic schoolmaster, instructing a rather slow-witted boy, says "This is a nut and that is a bolt. It is a long-established custom that the one goes inside the other, thus. If your forefathers, Wigglesworth, had been as stupid as you are, the human race would never have succeeded in procreating itself."

GID manifests such a stark contradiction between the felt self and the reality of the body that severe mental splitting seems to be indicated. A sense of reality based on an experience of the "self" as one having mental and physical attributes (rather than a mind in a body) develops from processes involving the linking and integration of experience, both internal and external. When integration is obstructed or compromised, mental bifurcation into twin-track functioning may occur, so that two different and completely contradictory perceptions of reality and the self can be entertained simultaneously. A split between material and psychic satisfaction develops.

The following case draws attention to such issues in relation to sexual reassignment surgery and is germane to the problem so vividly represented in "Colin's Story".

The patient, female, was referred to me at an NHS psychotherapy clinic: she complained of depression and of feeling persecuted and bullied by other patients at the gender clinic which she had been attending for some time. It turned out that the patient had had substantial hormonal treatment but had yet to undergo the surgery for genital change, and this had become the focus of her anxiety and depression. She was most convincing as a woman in voice and appearance: her bearing could hardly have been better represented than in the serene elegance of the cat in Colin's first picture. However, "she" had a penis whose fate was a matter of intense anxiety, and I found myself facing the difficult position of how to address this patient. I concluded that I was in the presence of a male who was contemplating the mutilation of his body in order to believe that he was a woman. He (she) reacted to the word "mutilation" with consternation and said, "I am certain I am 99.9% female", while adding "though not, of course, biologically". He then went on to tell me that it was only when he looked in the mirror that he was unable to deny the reality of his penis and that he was very fearful of the unknown outcome of submitting to surgery. The split in his thinking meant that he could only think of the surgery in relation to the fantasy of being female and the wish not to have a penis, but not in relation to what he was doing in reality to his real male body. His dilemma is admirably portrayed by the metamorphic sequences in the drawings of the cat's ever-receding tail. The patient wished for his penis to disappear but quailed at the thought of real surgical removal.

For this patient, threads of contact with reality remained. First in the mirror experience, which he described and again in the defeatism with which he contemplated his relationship with his partner, a bisexual man for whom he could never bear a child. Ultimately, it was his respect for reality that was causing him such pain and was, apparently, also a source of torment for other patients at the gender clinic who could not bear his agony. He spoke of a transsexual hierarchy: those who had had surgery, hostile and contemptuous of those who had not.

This case also supports Pfäfflin's view that sexuality *per se* is not a significant factor in the wish for gender change. What this man wanted above all was "to have a husband": someone to support and protect him. His was an unconditional and self-effacing love that made no demands of his partner. He anticipated and accepted without protest the possibility that his partner might one day want to leave him, in order to return to a woman and have children. The reality of this man's life was tragic. While he felt safer disguised as a woman, he remained vigilant and constantly afraid of being discovered to be male. It is as if he were trying to recreate an intra-uterine existence, his male gender enclosed in a female shell. His terror relates to fears for his own survival rather than to losing the object, and thoughts of suicide as the only way, ultimately, to find relief were also present.

Anxiety about genital ambiguity in intersex cases has a focus in the body, while those who suffer from GID fear for their viability and survival. Coates is persuaded that the suffering of those with GID is of a different order. The experience of separateness and therefore, separation anxiety, is removed when "being inside" serves as a regressive substitute for internalizing experience. However, the extreme vulnerability of this illusion is experienced as life-threatening.

6

Research, research politics, and clinical experience with transsexual patients

Friedemann Pfäfflin

When reflecting on the century since the publication of Freud's (1905d) *Three Essays on the Theory of Sexuality* (1905d), we are not far off the one-hundredth anniversary of the first sex reassignment surgery (SRS) performed in 1912. The term transsexualism did not exist in those days, and the phenomenon described by it was not mentioned in Freud's *Three Essays*. Yet none of all the sexual abnormalities mentioned in his book has hitherto attracted as much attention as transsexualism. Although the number of transsexuals is comparatively small, the challenge they pose is tremendous.

I start with my first clinical encounter with a transsexual patient (see also Pfäfflin, 1994, 2003) and then, embedded in a narrative of own experiences, add some general research data before turning to very few psychoanalytic findings.

First encounters

As a medical student I appreciated the opportunity to regularly assist a famous psychiatrist, Eberhard Schorsch, at the Department of Sex Research at Hamburg University Clinic. He saw the most extraordinary people who had committed serious crimes, in order to prepare psychiatric expert evaluations for courts. He enabled his patients to talk by being reserved, treading softly, and listening attentively. Although not a psychoanalyst, he was regarded by the courts, by lawyers, and by the public at large as *the* psychoanalytic forensic psychiatrist in the country because of his capacity to create insight into the motives for and circumstances of the patients' horrible deeds.

However, in the case of the first patient presenting transsexual symptoms whom I saw with him, his typical engaging reserve gave way to total passivity. The patient talked almost endlessly—without appearing to need a stimulus. It was as if he was allowed to talk into empty space, and he did not appear for the next session. When this same pattern of my mentor's passivity repeated itself with the second and third transsexual patient, I asked him about the reasons for his different behaviour with these patients. I recognized that I had strongly identified with the patients and what I perceived to be their feeling of being at a total loss because of the doctor's lack of response.

He explained that he could only marginally relate to the patients' wish for "sex change" and "not much could be done anyway". The University Clinic of Hamburg did not have the facilities to tackle this difficult problem. The patients might go to a clinic in Casablanca, Morocco, where SRS was offered in those days, or to one of the new gender identity clinics in the United States. He suggested that I should do a clinical attachment there, if I was interested. Following his advice, I spent several weeks at the Johns Hopkins University Gender Identity Clinic in Baltimore, Maryland, which, since 1965, had been the first US university clinic to carry out "sex change". Along with John Money and his co-workers, I was able to talk to a large number of patients who sought assessment, therapy, or follow-up. I was amazed to observe how openly patients with transsexual symptoms were received. I was also fascinated by the patients themselves and developed a great interest in sex research and gender issues. Later, back in Germany, I held a position as assistant under Schorsch.

By this time the situation within the Department for Sex Research had changed markedly. In a much-praised paper, Schorsch (1974) had characterized the "sex change operation as treatment without alternative" for transsexuals. As a consulting psychoanalyst, Burzig (unpublished manuscript, 1978; see also Burzig, 1982) saw transsexual patients in psychoanalytic interviews. Colleagues at the newly opened Department of Sexual Science at the University Clinic in Frankfurt am Main presented a survey on transsexualism, discussing, among general findings (from medicine as well as from psychoanalysis—for example, referring to Margaret Mahler and Otto Kernberg), the work of psychoanalysts who had seen patients with transvestite or transsexual symptoms (e.g. Haynal, 1974; Person & Ovesey, 1974a, 1974b; Schwöbel, 1960a; Socarides, 1970b; Stoller, 1968, 1975c; Thomä, 1957). Relying on this review, they compiled an "examination and treatment programme" for transsexuals that became, for a couple of years, the basic guide and point of orientation in the field in Germany (Sigusch, Meyenburg, & Reiche, 1978, 1979).

This programme begins with a list of 12 major criteria, which I found useful in parts but in others more discouraging—for example, at one point the patients are described as being "possessed by the desire for sex change" (a metaphor that calls to mind healing by prayer and casting out of devils rather than psychotherapy or any other medical procedure). This desire, it went on to say, can be "compulsive and endless". The patients refused psychotherapy, even hated it, and they were disgusted by the gender-specific characteristics of their bodies and often exhibited a "considerable diffusion of reality". "Nobody advocates gender specific matters more passionately than them." Criteria 9, 11, and 12 are most strongly formulated, excerpts of which are given here:

> (9) In medical conversation transsexuals appear to be cool, distanced and emotionless, rigid, unconcerned and unwilling to compromise, egocentric, coercive, fanatically obsessed and hemmed in, strangely uniform, standardised, stereotypical . . . the ability for introspection and transference are for the most part lacking. Confrontation and trial interpretations are often ineffective. Despite a frequently incessant description of his suffering, the patient shows almost no emotion. With his talkativeness, often marked by gestures and empty phrases, the patient seems stereotypical, monotonous, superficial.
>
> (11) Human relationships of transsexuals are seriously disturbed as their ability to empathise and to bond with others is considerably lacking. Transsexuals tend either to idealise or to belittle other people strongly. Polarisations such as 'all or nothing', 'properly or not at all', 'now or never', govern every single area of experience and behaviour in transsexuals lives.

(12) If transsexuals have the impression that they are not being supported or are being hindered in their wish for a sex change, they often exhibit reactions ranging from irritability and aggressiveness to extreme moodiness. All transsexuals exhibit a tendency towards psychotic collapse under stress, in situations of crisis. Suicide and self mutilation attempts which have to be taken seriously may then occur.

Formulations and static statements such as these are, in my view, akin to the final "laying to rest" of a person, the refusal to give any more chances. The way patients were described seemed to be owed to the terminology of psychopathology of the nineteenth century. (It was only 18 years later that the first author of this examination and treatment programme renounced these statements—Sigusch, 1997). It did not correspond with what I had witnessed with patients in Baltimore and only partially with what I had experienced with patients in Hamburg. Without doubt there were individual patients who could be characterized in this way, but it appeared to me that not enough attention was being paid either to the situational factors in the treatment or to the personal accounts of those providing it.

In particular, I was preoccupied by Burzig's comments at the Thirteenth Conference of the German Society for Sexual Research in October 1978, when he said that his experiences in psychoanalytic interviews confirmed the passages just quoted. He had also experienced the patients as "cool, distanced and emotionless, rigid, unconcerned and unwilling to compromise, egocentric, coercive, fanatically obsessed and hemmed in, strangely uniform, standardized, stereotypical, monotonous, and superficial" (Burzig, 1982, p. 852). At the following conference of this society in October 1982, Reiche, also a psychoanalyst who had cooperated in the development of the Frankfurt examination and treatment programme, referred to the patients as "monsters" (see also Reiche, 1984).

Both Reiche's and Burzig's work reflected some of the tension engendered in the discussion of so-called "sex changes", which, among psychiatrists, continually lead to controversy (e.g. Boss, 1950–51; Kubie & Mackie, 1968; Mitscherlich, 1950–51; Mitscherlich et al., 1950–51a, 1950–51b; Springer, 1981). There was a tendency towards an all-or-nothing approach, which was immediately declared the characteristic of the pathological organization of the patients. The pros and cons of surgical procedure had become a shibboleth in specialist discussions rather than with the patients themselves, who represented a much wider spectrum. Alongside patients adamant in their demands for surgery and apparently unprepared to consider any other course of action were those open to psychotherapeutic work or who took up appropriate suggestions without any great resistance and were extremely sceptical of the "surgical solution".

The Frankfurt criteria, along with Burzig's negative catalogue and Reiche's "monsters", caused a strong personal reaction and led to my hypothesis that transsexual symptoms are a creative defence mechanism (Pfäfflin, 1983). Such an explanation seemed necessary, as it was so difficult to persuade analytically active colleagues to treat patients with transsexual symptoms. Let me give one example: A female patient, very motivated towards psychotherapy, had contacted me. As I did not have an immediate empty space, she tried to find a treatment place with five colleagues. In some of the initial interviews, when she mentioned her transsexual symptoms, she was asked unconditionally to agree not to undergo any hormonal or surgical procedures until after the treatment was over. But as physical treatment was her firm intention, she could, and would, not agree to this condition. In other interviews she was advised to wait first for the results of somatic treatment (which had not even begun) before getting in touch again. The third variation consisted of referring her back to me, from where her search for treatment had originated, because "he deals with this sort of problem". She was only able to find a place in treatment after an interview in which she, following my advice, did not mention her transsexual symptoms at all. After several sessions she gained enough confidence to reveal her central problem, and at this point the therapist immediately terminated the treatment.

If there is any room for doubt as to the conviction to belong to the other sex—psychoanalysts might conceive of this conviction as an identity resistance (Erikson, 1968; Pfäfflin, 1994)—these doubts cannot surface in the mind of the patient as long as the psychoanalyst is preoccupied with them and does not provide a safe space in which the patient can reorganize his or her defensive patterns.

I felt in identification with the demoted position of the patient and read Burzig's (1982) and Reiche's (1984) lectures over and over again, now considerably revised for publication, in order to recall that these authors, quite apart from the statements that even today still seem derogatory, had also expressed a great deal of sympathy for the patients in their countertransference. Reiche described how strongly he sometimes felt the pull of empathy to the patients' wishes—so much so, in fact, that he could even come to wish it himself, carried away by the mood of the moment. In a similar way Burzig had written that

> more or less consciously we develop an empathy for how terrible it must be for the experience of one's own identity to feel that one does not really belong to either gender, to live in no man's land or—genetically speaking—in the advances. This empathy could motivate us to "bring out" the patients and to end their suffering through the provision of another "uniform". [Burzig, 1982, p. 854]

It was only many years later that I asked myself why I had been so identified with the demoted position of the patients, and the hypothetical answer I found is that it must have to do with my first name, Friedemann [man of peace] and its parody. When, as a pre-school child, I was in a rage for whatever reason, my many brothers and sisters liked to tease me by calling me *Kriegsfrau* [woman of war]. Retrospectively, I suppose, this is the biographical background that has stimulated my interest in transsexualism and in persons unsure of their gender identity. The attack on one's own gender identity touches a sensitive spot, and I could empathize with those feeling not at home in their body.

Since my first encounter in 1971, I have seen and accompanied more than 1,000 persons with transsexual symptoms for shorter or longer periods and at various frequencies, from twice-a-year to four-times-a-week in a face-to-face setting, and I have followed the development of quite a few of them for 20 or more—some even for 30—years. With most of them, the most intensive treatment episodes were at the very beginning, before they took the decision to have hormonal and surgical treatment in addition. Sometimes psychotherapy intensified when the somatic treatment had started. In a number of cases the most intensive and fruitful episodes of psychodynamic treatment started only many years after SRS. Only one of the patients did I, at the beginning of my clinical career, treat four times per week in the classical setting on the couch, because he insisted on this setting, but this was a mistake. The patient regressed rapidly and committed a serious suicide attempt, demanding in-patient treatment in a distant surgical rehabilitation unit for several months.

Terminology and politics

Only two years before the first SRS was performed in 1912, Magnus Hirschfeld (1910), a protagonist of the homosexual liberation movement, coined the term "transvestism". In the first decade of the twentieth century some noblemen with close connections to the German Kaiser Wilhelm II were accused of homosexual acts, then still a felony. One faction, oriented towards an idealized Greek type of socially well-adjusted lifestyle, therefore feared the failure of its attempts to abolish criminal sanctions against gay men if homosexuality included so-called effeminate styles, drag queens, fags, and so on. Hirschfeld (1910) reacted by publishing a two-volume monograph with the title *Die Transvestiten* [The Transvestites], thus creating a new category separate from homosexuality and no longer embarrassing for the gay liberation movement. The book contained biographies of people, many of whom would now be called transsexuals. The term "transvestite" remained the leading term for cross-dressing men, and sometimes also for cross-dressing women, until the 1960s, regardless of whether these persons changed their roles only temporarily or wished for permanent hormonal and surgical sex reassignment. In 1923 Hirschfeld, in passing, also used the term *Transsexualismus* [transsexualism] for the first time. In many publications, Cauldwell (1949) is credited to have invented this term. Benjamin (1966), who published the first monograph on the topic, even claimed to have invented it. While Cauldwell was strongly opposed to SRS, Benjamin had met Hirschfeld frequently and certainly had learned from him, including the word transsexualism (Pfäfflin, 1997).

That this term became a category of its own was mainly due to the availability of hormonal and surgical sex reassignment. The first prospective study on transsexualism was started in 1963 in Sweden (Walinder, 1967), followed by studies at the Gender Identity Clinic at the Johns Hopkins University Clinic in Baltimore, established in 1965. To justify medical treatments, you need, first of all, a proper medical diagnosis. Transvestism was not suitable for this purpose because it implied such a wide range of behaviours, some of which were still criminalized in many countries in those days. Harry Benjamin's (1966) monograph *The Transsexual Phenomenon* demonstrated that transsexualism was a medical problem that had to be tackled. This was a time when sexual research was expanding rapidly. Its cornerstone had been sexual pathology and forensics, developed in Austria and Germany in the nineteenth century in the cooperation between law and psychiatry. Modern post-Second-World-War sexology built on the sociological studies of Kinsey, Pomeroy, and Martin (1948, 1953) as the first pillar; on the study of intersex and transsexual conditions initiated by John Money in Baltimore and with new gender identity clinics shooting up like mushrooms in many places, as the second pillar; and, finally, with physiological research on sexual functioning and couple therapy, initiated by Masters and Johnson (1966, 1970), as the third pillar.

In 1980, the diagnosis of transsexualism was included in the *Diagnostic and Statistical Manual of the American Psychiatric Association.* In 1991, the *International Classification of Diseases,* edited by the World Health Organization, adopted it and closely connected the diagnosis with hormonal and surgical treatment, as if the diagnosis automatically implied one specific form of treatment. Three years later, in 1994, the diagnosis was deleted from DSM–IV and replaced by the more general diagnosis of Gender Identity Disorder (GID).

The medicalization of gender issues provoked a countermovement: the movement of transgenderists, initiated by Virginia Prince (1978), originally a transvestite, permanently living in the female role yet not wishing to get rid of her male genitalia. Transgenderism soon became the umbrella term for transvestites and transsexuals. At that time, "trans" referred to transformation and crossing. In the 1990s a new meaning of "trans" emerged in the now widespread use of the word transgender, with "trans" now alluding to transgression, going beyond the binary divide of the sexes. Sociologists Richard Ekins and Dave King are going even further and suggest a fourth meaning of transgenderism. Referring to ethno-methodological research as developed by Kessler and McKenna (1985), Foucault, and themselves, they posit that it is no longer possible to argue that sex is nature and gender is socio-cultural. Instead, both come to be seen as socio-cultural, and the binary itself a social construction. They define the task of a "scientific 'transgender studies' to map the various constructions of transgender phenomena in terms of their origins, developments, interrelations and consequences" (Ekins & King, 2006; see also Ekins, 1997; Ekins & King, 1996). They situate their theory, methodology, and research techniques within the social interactionist (constructionist) view of science put forward by George Herbert Mead (Strauss, 1964) and Herbert Blumer (1969), a tradition that has been restated in more contemporary terms by Anselm Strauss (1993) and Robert Prus (1997).

Medical research, biology, and politics

Medical research is usually looking for causes to be able to offer causal treatment. This is also true for the history of transsexualism. Initially, chromosomal and hormonal aberrations were sought for to explain transsexualism. When this failed, prenatal hormonal conditions were explored, using rat and other experiments to hypothesize early imprinting processes on the human brain. It is obvious that the rat, lacking self-reflection, is not a good model for transsexualism. Now, neurobiology is the hit, and the scarce findings from six post-mortem brains of transsexuals serve as argument to locate differences in the Bed Nucleus of the area striata of the hypothalamus (Kruijver, 2004; Zhou, Hofman, Gooren, & Swaab, 1995). Some 25 years ago we had to struggle with the short-lived hypothesis that an H–Y-antigen deficit would be the moving force of gender identity development. In the United Kingdom, the Gender Identity Research and Education Society (GIRES) is one of the most outspoken and active protagonists of the conviction that transsexualism is biologically founded.

> The current medical viewpoint, based on the most up-to-date scientific research, is that Gender Dysphoria, which in its extreme manifestation is known as transsexualism, is strongly associated with a neuro-developmental condition of the brain. Small areas of the brain are known to be distinctly different in 'males' and 'females' in the population generally. In those experiencing severe Gender Dysphoria, one of these areas has been shown to become sex-reversed in early development and is, therefore, incongruent with the other sex characteristics. Sex differentiation of the brain is imperfectly understood, but it is believed to be associated with hormones impacting on the developing brain in an atypical way. [GIRES, 2004]

As in the history of homosexuality, there seems to be a zeal for a biological explanation that may, at the same time, serve to justify and to ennoble the condition as "natural", as if this would solve all other psychosocial issues inherent in it.

Children and adolescents

Another track of research is the observation of the development of children and adolescents displaying cross-gender behaviour at a young age. As many adult persons with transsexual symptoms claim to have felt different from the onset of their memories ("I have always felt like a woman, as long as I can remember"—a remarkable statement for a, retrospectively, 4-year-old boy), Stoller and Green were happy to study these children, of whom they first thought that they would finally turn out to become transsexuals in adulthood. This was obviously not the case, and the vast majority finally ended up as heterosexual or homosexual individuals, which caused Robert Green (1987b) to describe the "Sissy Boy Syndrome" as a precursor of homosexuality. Expanded clinical research with adolescents suggests that cross-gender behaviour in that life span seems rather fixated in a large number of cases (Cohen-Kettenis & Pfäfflin, 2003; DiCeglie & Freedman, 1998; Zucker & Bradley, 1995).

Legislation and administrative provisions for sex reassignment

Switzerland and Germany were the first countries to allow legal name and sex change in individual cases in the 1930s and 1940s. These cases did not draw much public attention; they were solved more or less in silence. Thus it was possible not only to change one's legal status *ex nunc* (from the time of the surgery) but also *ex tunc* (retrospectively from birth onwards). After the Second World War, legal sex change in Europe was much more complicated. The argument of the invariability of the sex of a person was again strong in many countries that derived their law from Napoleon's *Code Civil* of 1804. In those countries the birth certificate is the source for all other documents. Therefore it is essential to change the sex in this document to endow a person with the full rights of the new gender. In the Anglo-American tradition it was easier to adopt a new first name, yet often not the full rights of the new gender.

The first specific law for sex reassignment for transsexuals was passed in 1972 by Sweden, and it was the trailblazer for all consecutive laws and administrative solutions in other countries. Germany followed in 1980, allowing for a change of the first name to make it easier for the person to pass in the new gender role even without any form of treatment, and for the full change of the legal status from male to female and vice versa after SRS. In 1981 in Austria an administrative solution was implemented. Italy passed a similar law in 1982, followed by The Netherlands in 1985, Turkey in 1988, and Finland in 2003. Some countries resisted for quite a while and had to be sentenced by the European Court of Human Rights (ECHR) in Strasbourg—for example, France in 1992, and ten years later the United Kingdom. The United Kingdom had won its case in some previous decisions of the ECHR and had refused persons after SRS to marry in their new gender role until the ECHR on 11 July 2002 delivered its judgment in the case of *Goodwin v The United Kingdom* and *I v The United Kingdom* (*Human Rights Law Journal, 23*: 72–85), thus paving the way for the Gender Recognition Act of 1 July 2004. All of the more than 40 member states of the ECHR now accept full legal sex change. Belgium goes even further. It still registers the sex of a child at birth, but when it comes to marriage, this is not an essential. Any adult can get married to another adult, no matter whether this is a person of the same or the opposite sex, a person with an intersex condition, a homosexual, or a transsexual. Thus, as regards marriage, specific regulations for sex change are not needed for transsexuals in Belgium.

Results of SRS

In psychoanalytic literature it is often maintained that the outcome of SRS is unfavourable and a mutilation; that the zeal of the patients for perfection never comes to an end; that many patients commit suicide postoperatively; and that the number of regrets is high. A favourite statement in this literature is that a sex reassignment will never be complete because, for example, the chromosomes cannot be changed, or, as some authors have formulated, a postoperative male-to-female transsexual (MFT) will be nothing but a castrated man.

Together with my colleague Astrid Junge, I did a meta-analysis of all follow-up studies after SRS published between 1961 and 1991, including only samples with at least five or more postoperative patients. It comprised 76 follow-up studies and 8 reviews comprising a total of about 1,000–1,500 MFT and 500 FMT (Pfäfflin & Junge, 1992b, 1998). The results were encouraging and much more favourable than expected. They can be summarized as follows: sex reassignment treatment is effective. Positive effects clearly outweigh undesired effects. There are seven factors promoting a good outcome: (1) the patient's continuous contact with a treatment centre, (2) cross-gender living or real-life experience, (3) cross-hormone treatment, (4) counselling and psychotherapy, (5) surgery, (6) quality of surgery, and (7) legal acknowledgement of sex change. The large number of hitherto published follow-up studies confirms these findings.

On average, the results are better in female-to-male transsexuals (FMT). In FMT, regrets amounted to less than 1%, in male-to-females (MFT) to 1.5% (Pfäfflin, 1992). Suicide attempts and suicides are much more frequent in preoperative transsexuals than after SRS. Personally I have met some ten patients who retrospectively regretted the sex change, three of whom I had referred to the surgeon myself years before. They were not reproachful; on the contrary, all of them emphasized the inevitability of their former decision and said it had saved their life.

Returning to psychoanalysis

Psychoanalytic and psychodynamic treatment (without or including certain parameters—see also Meyenburg, 1992) may also be a means to survive for a person with transsexual symptoms. Yet the number of such reports is astonishingly small, given the great theoretical challenge transsexualism poses to psychoanalysis. I would be surprised if anybody could present more than 30 full psychoanalytic case reports (for some recent ones see Gutowski, 2000; Quinodoz, 1998, 2002; Stein, 1995). Initially psychoanalysts were driven by the interest to understand the condition much more than by the interest to understand and thus support the patient. Some analysts may have pursued the goal to liberate the patient from his or her wish for a sex change, and initially I shared this goal, knowing quite well that it is a serious impediment for psychoanalytic treatment when the therapist has such goals in mind.

What do we learn from psychoanalytic writings about transsexuals? Primarily a lot of theory and generalizations, often derived from a single case study—sometimes even from an early dropout (e.g. Greenson, 1968). Person and Ovesey (1974a, 1974b), who have contributed much to the understanding of transsexualism, wrote: "To know one is to know them all", and I was happy to read that Ethel Person now cringes when rereading her old text (Person, 2001). The generalizations are already expressed in the titles of books (e.g. Désirat, *Die transsexuelle Frau* [*The* transsexual woman], 1985), in headings of chapters (e.g. Lothstein, 1983: "*The* female transsexual") or titles of articles (e.g. Chiland, 2000: "*The* psychoanalyst and *the* transsexual patient"; Herold, 2004: "Psychoanalyse *der* Transsexualität"; see also the subtitle of Quinodoz, 2002: "An example of general validity"). Relying on one patient and only rarely on a larger number, transsexuals are, by a number of authors, all classified as psychotic, borderline, perverse, or, not perverse but blissfully symbiotic, delusional, narcissistic, trapped in a homosexual emergency reaction, and so forth. In 1991, Oppenheimer wrote on the first page of her paper in the *International Journal of Psycho-Analysis* with the heading "The Wish for Sex Change: A Challenge to Psychoanalysis?":

> Transsexuals are pervaded by an obsession, an invasive concern about their bodily transformation. They exhibit neither perverse transvestism nor manifest psychosis. They are distrustful, they lie readily, they see the difference between the sexes in a stereotyped way, they trivialize their problems and they completely disavow homosexuality. [Oppenheimer, 1991, p. 221]

None of these statements would have been confirmed if the author had ever seen a large-enough number of persons suffering from transsexual symptoms. What she states is but a compilation of prejudices. Similarly, the abstract of Chiland's (2000, p. 21; see also Chiland, 2003) paper in the same journal reads as follows: "In particular, they are totally focused on the body and on their intention of securing sex reassignment by hormonal and surgical treatments, so that they rule out the involvement of any psychic element. . . ." She concludes that transsexualism is a narcissistic disorder in which the constitution of the self has been profoundly impaired. That is stating the obvious: when one does not feel at home in one's own body, that should, indeed, be a sign of a narcissistic problem.

I do not want to ridicule psychoanalytic writings on transsexualism as I would have to include my only own case report on a high-frequency long-term psychoanalytic treatment (Pfäfflin, 1994), which identified separation anxiety as one of the main problems of the patient described and emphasized the identity resistance and the alloautoplastic intersection between patient and therapist. Others have focused on a number of other preoedipal and oedipal anxieties. More or less successfully, we all apply the theoretical concepts we prefer. Sometimes they may be trivial and do no harm to the patient; at other times they may be helpful; and, finally, they may miss the inner and outer reality of the patient, and that usually results in dropouts.

One of the theories that outraged me most at the beginning of my psychoanalytic career was not a psychoanalytic but an economic one. In 1981, I visited a sex research congress in Venezuela, and a colleague presented a paper explaining the increase in numbers of transsexuals in Venezuela with the extreme poverty that drove people for reasons of mere survival into the sex business. I heavily opposed his view, and did so again, when I was confronted with similar findings in Thailand. After having met larger numbers of transsexuals from these countries, I had to acknowledge that there was some truth in it. This, again, should not be generalized. It is only mentioned to caution us against the belief that transsexuals all suffer from the same psychopathology. As Limentani had already correctly stated in 1979, transsexualism is the final common pathway of a great variety of different starting points.

My present clinical practice I have described in more detail for a non-psychoanalytically oriented readership of mental health professionals in the *Handbook of Clinical Sexuality*, edited by Steve Levine (Pfäfflin, 2003). In two decades I have not met a single person with transsexual symptoms who uncompromisingly demanded hormonal treatment or SRS. This has certainly to do with my attitude towards these procedures, which I find as useful as psychoanalysis, telling the patient in the intake interview that he or she will undoubtedly be able to reach this goal if they so wish. I then offer my support in widening their scope and exploring their inner and outer worlds. The many facets of life I then encounter in this field, even after more than three decades, keep fascinating me.

Concluding remarks

After reviewing this chapter for publication and considering the discussion that followed its original presentation, I feel that some further clarifications would be appropriate. Peter Fonagy, whose comments on my chapter I very much appreciate, highlights the messages I wanted to convey. A person presenting as a "trans" person wants to be recognized and acknowledged in her own right, including her suffering, her social circumstances, and the visions she has of how she could live best. As psychoanalysts, we engage in long-term and in-depth interactions with patients, identifying with their views of themselves and confronting them with what we know about psychosocial development and functioning in general. What can be learned from the treatment of one patient may be helpful when treating a second patient in similar distress. At other times, however, experience with one patient may not be applicable to another person or may even be misleading, even though their suffering seems to be very similar. A patient may choose and profit from more practical solutions as well as from psychodynamic insight, although as psychoanalysts we might prefer to rank insight higher than acting in and acting out. By broadening our perspectives and by acknowledging that there is more than one option in tackling psychic suffering, the chances that patients can make use of psychoanalytic treatment will certainly increase.

Peter Fonagy poses a number of questions, on which I will comment briefly.

To "distinguish the identity aspect of sexuality from the pleasurable, raunchy components" is difficult. In orgasmic intercourse these two aspects cannot usually be distinguished: they fuse, as do the two persons involved. To give an example:

> A patient of mine, a former FMT with incomplete SRS—that is, he had had testosterone treatment for years, breast reduction surgery, as well as hysterectomy, but no phalloplasty, and had been married as a man for more than a decade—fell in love with his male Italian teacher, who knew nothing about his history. They decided to go to bed with each other just like any other homosexual couple might have done. It was only then that the Italian friend realized that there was no second penis, and they decided to have sexual intercourse, an overwhelming experience for my former patient who enthusiastically told me about it. When I asked him whether this experience did not call his male identity into question, his answer was "no", and he added: "We both had a penis, the penis belonged to both of us." In no way did he experience the encounter as a traditional heterosexual encounter and himself thrown back into the female position. On the contrary, he

> experienced himself as a man engaging in a homosexual activity. Accordingly, when sexually interacting with his wife, he experienced himself as a man engaging in heterosexual activities, not in lesbian ones, regardless of whether they used a dildo or not.

The example illustrates that gender identity and sexual excitement, although developmentally closely linked, do not merge but can be clearly differentiated. Gender identity is, supposedly, the organizing factor of any sexual behaviour.

Sexual behaviour of persons with transsexual symptoms shows the same diversity as is found in the population at large. Some of these persons live a totally asexual life, others are moderately active or on an average level, and others still are preoccupied with sexual desires, thoughts, and activities and tend to sexualize most of their stronger affects, as is usually found in perversions (Goldberg, 1995). Gender identity and sexual orientation—as bisexual, homosexual, or heterosexual—are interlinked by common roots yet largely independent of each other when fully organized in adulthood. In my view the variance mainly depends on the structural level of the personality organization of the individual. The more sexualization there is and the greater the acting out of perverse impulses, the less stable the gender identity (Schorsch, Galedary, Haag, Hauch, & Lohse, 1990). This holds true generally and is not specific for persons with transsexual symptoms.

I doubt that transsexualism can tell us much about "normal" sexuality. If anything, it may tell us that sexuality may be more variable over the life span than we would normally have expected. It is usually assumed that gender identity and sexual orientation are fixed around puberty—some authors might give a somewhat earlier or later date. Just as there are homosexuals with a very late coming out, so some transsexuals have a late coming out: at the age of 50, or even later. Often neither they nor their family or close friends would have expected such a development. Thus, gender identity as well as identity represent "sameness in process" rather than fixed states. Some of these individuals with a late coming-out surprise themselves and others as regards the flexibility of their sexual desires and behaviours. This is also true for the small percentage of those who regret prior SRS and return to their original gender role, sometimes, yet not always, again reversing sexual behaviour patterns. In my understanding, the modifications of sexual behaviour in the course of a transsexual career seem to be secondary to the underlying gender identity problem.

As regards the present neuroscientific reductionism, I have already mentioned the position of the Gender Identity Research and Education Society (GIRES, 2004), the agency that most outspokenly posits a neurobiological causation of transsexualism. This is the fashion of the day for many psychological problems, and although its protagonists may want to preclude alternative psychological or social explanations, they will certainly fall short of this aim in the long run. As pointed out in my chapter, there have been other biomedical theories pursuing the same aim. New techniques of investigation usually challenge all prior explanations of whatever phenomenon and claim to have found the philosopher's stone. One might take this with composure. To give a very peripheral example, not directly linked with neuroscience but with endocrinology: it is generally accepted knowledge that the male sex hormone testosterone enhances sexual arousal much more than the female sex hormones. It is therefore no surprise that some FMTs experience more sexual arousal when starting testosterone treatment, but this does not hold true by any means for all FMTs.

When administering female sex hormones to MFTs, one would expect the opposite: that is, inhibition of sexual arousal. I have often observed the converse. Some MFTs who had hardly any sexual interest as long as they were living in the male gender role reacted with a remarkable enhancement of sexual arousal after having started female sex hormone treatment. This is counter to endocrinological expectations and can, in my view, only be explained by psychological mechanisms. When living in the female gender role, getting female sex hormones, and growing breasts, MFTs accept themselves much more than before, no matter whether they are already accepted by others in their new gender role, and this makes them much more open and susceptible to sexual stimuli.

To return to neuroscience: if the number and size of neurons in any area of the brain decides whether or not a person becomes a transsexual, how does this account for the few patients who clearly were transsexuals but, later in life, regretted their decision for SRS and returned to their original gender role? It would be much too easy—and, incidentally, unsubstantiated—to claim that they had not been "true" transsexuals. I have talked to some of these individuals quite extensively and followed them up for longer periods. They spoke much more about the conditions of their growing up than they had ever done before. The same is true for transsexuals who do not regret SRS. They no longer have to fight for acknowledgement. They are much freer to look into their own histories, and some of them produce rich psychodynamic material. Collecting such stories will certainly reveal a wealth of knowledge about psychosocial influences and may contribute to our understanding of the moving forces behind the desire for SRS and the turning points of decision making in pursuit of this aim.

Commentary

Peter Fonagy

The first lesson in Pfäfflin's chapter is a historical one: the issue of transsexuality as resolvable by surgical procedure is about as old as psychoanalysis. Second, and hardly surprising, the mental health community has had considerable difficulty in accommodating to this problem, with the expectable splits and categorical—all good/all bad—thinking. It is neither surprising nor necessarily regrettable that psychoanalysts experience the world much the same way as any-one else. They react to "difference" with predictable anxieties and appropriate primitive defences. Only those who idealize the profes-sion claim that we can do more. The history that Pfäfflin delineates for us makes it clear that we are influenced by our cultural context in our appraisal of psychological problems not significantly less than are those who come to these issues without our training.

A further lesson concerns the value of sustained experience. As psychoanalysts, we have a significant handicap in developing a world view imposed by the length and intensity of our treatment. Our encounters with individuals are intensive and long-term, and this has many advantages. On the debit side is the practical fact that it precludes us from seeing a large number of individuals with similar problems. Pfäfflin's experience is based on having seen many hundreds of cases. Most psychoanalysts can only see a handful and are forced to generalize, often overgeneralize, from this tiny sample to the whole population. Much can be said about this problem that goes considerably beyond the topic of sexual deviation. The most important lesson, however, implicit in the chapter is that psychoanalytic clinicians do not have the tools or the conceptual framework to integrate experience beyond the single case. We need perhaps urgently to develop ways in which we could effectively combine our collective experiences with different types of patients by more standard reporting of the cases that we see, or through some other means.

More specifically, we learn about humility from Pfäfflin's chapter. We learn not just that our expectations of negative outcome from SRS appear largely unfounded, but also that we understand little about the causes of transsexualism and that working with half-baked ideas can sometimes do harm, not simply little good. Humility is also perhaps the appropriate reaction to the potency of the economic forces that can drive individuals in Third-World countries working in the sex industry to self mutilation. Our society of wealth can afford to put self-agency at the top of a motivational hierarchy. All too often we forget the privileged positions we occupy. Humility is also called for in relation to the expectations that individuals with transsexual wishes have of their therapists as well as of their medical carers. The humility counteracts the destructiveness of overvalued ideas.

Perhaps the most important lesson is one that pervades this volume: that knowledge and understanding of the individual has tremendous value, requires very special skills, and is of enormous benefit. The rules of thinking and rules of evidence required are, however, completely different from those that the explication of general causal mechanisms entail. It is not that the former are not causal accounts. The very nature of thinking about someone automatically entails identifying the reasons for their actions. When considering clinical problems rather than individuals with a problem, the rules of evidence are distinct: perhaps no more exacting, but certainly different. Intimate interpersonal interaction is driven by spontaneity, intuition, and parallel processes, while understanding of causal mechanisms in relation to a particular problem rather than a particular human being demands a linear systematic, for want of a better word, less romantic, more obsessional approach.

An issue that appears in several chapters, particularly chapter four by Richard Friedman, points to the need to distinguish the identity aspect of sexuality from the pleasurable, raunchy components. The close involvement of sexual pleasure with gender identity often conflates our attempts at conceptualizing problems such as transsexualism. Several questions, however, seem to require further elaboration: (1) What is the relationship between these two facets of belonging to a gender group? Perhaps it would be helpful to elaborate that the sexuality of the transsexual as sexuality is a major but by no means the only way of actualizing one's gender. (2) What, if anything, does transsexualism tell us about "normal" sexuality? About the nature of sexual pleasure as we commonly experience it? Are the modifications of experience of sexuality associated with transsexualism material or incidental? A secondary consequence of an underlying broader problem of gender identity? (3) Given that we face a period of neuroscientific reductionism that reveals the dualistic character of all our thinking, the zeal for a biological account appears to preclude a social explanation. Yet the brain, the organ of the mind, is constructed by evolution to come to maturity in a social context.

7

Drive and affect in perverse actions

Rainer Krause

Some general thoughts about perversions

Within the thinking and writing about perversion, two perspectives, which are not mutually exclusive, can be distinguished. On the one hand, perverse creations could be regarded as creative play forms of human life, which are in no way concerned with either the courts or therapy. Kernberg (1995) has shown that sadomasochistic fantasies are an important part of normal love relations. Much creative production is closely related to perverse acts, as Chasseguet-Smirgel (1985) has worked out. Perverse behaviour is so widespread and at the same time kept so secret that it is not surprising that in most epidemiological studies it does not even register (Schepanck, 1987). From that perspective, modern epidemiologists have given up the term altogether, talking about paraphilias instead admitting that the prevalence rate must be very high because the commercial market is overabundant (Sass, Wittchen, & Zaudig, 1996, p. 595).

On the other hand, most experts agree in that perversions represent a severe disturbance, with links to psychosis, fragmentation, and alienation (Khan, 1979). Again, Chasseguet-Smirgel (1983) considers perversion as an indicator for severe pathology, first at the level of the individual but also at the level of society, relating the amount of perversion to the collapse of the law that should be embedded in a culture through the internalization of a loving yet powerful father counteracting the infantile incestuous mother–child universe. Indeed, after years of treating such patients I can say that very often the perverse enactment is the major stronghold against the laws of treatment and at the same time against change. The perverse universe is often re-enacted in the treatment without the conscious knowledge of the therapist. One patient was in treatment for his "depression" for three years without ever mentioning his severe perverse constructions. Seeing me, as his second analyst, he began after a year to talk about bits of these constructions, talking very contemptuously about the lady therapist to whom he had lied all the time without realizing that he was breaking all rules and laws of treatment. He had asked me for a consultation knowing that I had a reputation for the treatment of perversions. Nevertheless, he lied to me also. Of course, the term "lying" is not suitable for the process because—as I will argue—patients will not be able to renounce these secret constructions before they can be sure that the world at large—that is, the analyst—has something better to offer. This is nearly impossible, because hope based on a minimum of idealization is counteracted by secret scripts of enacting contempt and disgust to regulate the density of cathexis and to keep the oedipal figures powerless. I will argue that such constellations are very frequent, and usually they go unnoticed. In order to understand the structural commonalities of perverse solutions disregarding the phenomenology of perverse behaviour, it is helpful to use our research knowledge about affects and drives.

Perverse behaviour and structures

As my purpose is to derive the idea of structure from a specific relation between drive and affect, I present some basics about affect, then the drives, and, finally, on the relation between them, relying on our earlier work (Krause, 1983, 1991; Krause, Steimer-Krause, & Ullrich, 1992). Then, with this knowledge, I analyse a perverse act that I consider easy to understand, on the basis of the processes that are part of this action. Finally, I return to the definition of perversion, its origin and treatment.

Definition of affect

In the clinical praxis we distinguish four different contexts in which the concept of affect is used:

1. Affects are described as derivates of drive activity as signals of *Lust/Unlust* [pleasure/unpleasure] (Freud, 1915c, *G.S.*, p. 9). From their biological functioning and neuroanatomical architecture they are reinforcement and reward systems that are associated with the terminal acts of a drive process. They are phylogenetically much older than the affect system to which they are related only loosely (Panksepp, 1998). We will use the German terms *Lust* and *Unlust* for these affective signals. *Lust* and affects can be relatively freely combined. There is, for example, fear–*Lust*, disgust–*Lust*, anger–*Lust*, and happiness–*Unlust*, curiosity–*Unlust*, just to mention a few paradoxical combinations. These combinations—especially disgust–*Lust*—are essential for the understanding of perverse structures.
2. We speak of traumatic affects that are supposed to indicate system breakdowns. They are mobilized when the cognitive affective processing no longer functions.
3. We speak of affects as signals between structures, such as shame as an experiential sign that the "ego" receives from the "ego-ideal" as a measuring agent for transgression of rules.
4. We speak of affects as specific monitoring systems for object relations.

This affect system is built as parallel monitoring system that can be pinned down to six different modules in one person (Krause, 2000).

The motoric expressive system, the physiological system, the nonexpressive motoric system are embedded in the body. They operate within it without necessarily having any mental representation. On the representational side we have the perception of the body processes, especially the physiology that is called interoception, the language about affects, and, finally, a cognitive frame that is specific for each affect. These different systems can be described as modules that are, under normal conditions, only loosely connected. If two persons interact, this adds up to twelve interacting modules. It is essential to understand the social implications of that system: that the interdependence of these modules is higher between two persons than within one subject, allowing the understanding of the social partner. Because of space limitations I will mention only two of the modules: namely the *motoric expressive module* and the internal representation of the specific affect as a cognitive frame.

Within the periphery of the body (for example the face and the voice) a set of signs has developed in phylogenesis, carrying meaning. The signs symbolize joy, anger, disgust, sadness, contempt, curiosity, and fear. Other persons seeing or hearing these signs make inferences on the internal state of the sign emitters, which are interculturally similar. So specific innervations of the zygomaticus major and the ring muscle around the eye with a certain temporal pattern are interpreted in 98% of all cases as indicative of joyful movement towards an object.

This does not mean that the subject is necessarily feeling like that. The ability to innervate these signs and the ability to read them have coevolved in phylogeny during the same time period. In the context of our discussion this means that from 3 months of age on, humans can decipher the meaning of these signs via direct links from the thalamus to the amygdala long before there is any self-reflective awareness (Endres de Oliveira & Krause, 1989); on the contrary, there is evidence that the self-constituting feelings are determined through the affective signs of others (Fonagy, Gergely, Jurist, & Target, 2002).

The affective process is mentally represented as an *episode* with the experiencing subject: an object and a specific interaction between the two of them. The different affects are represented through a specific mental representation of an interaction between subject and object. This protocognitive frame is usually not conscious but is nevertheless active from early life on (Bischof, 1989; Riedl, 1981). It depicts mentally the pool of object relations that came to be highly relevant for survival in the phylogenesis of mankind. In nonpsychoanalytic theories of affects they are called "core relations" (Lazarus, 1993).

In the following I describe some of the protocognitive frames of affects. With *anger*, an object hinders important goals of the subject. The subject feels equal or superior in power. The proposition describing the episode is: "You, object, go away, I will stay!" *Fear* has the same parameters as anger, but the subject feels that the object

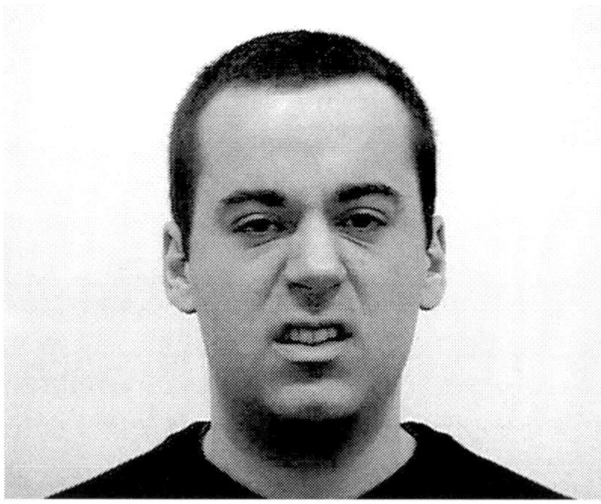

Figure 7.1

is more powerful than the subject. The proposition is: "You, object, stay, I will go away immediately." With *sadness* a former benevolent object is missing, and the proposition is: "You, object, come back to me." Anger and fear are very close in physiology, and the protocognitive structure leads to frequent flipping between the states. Only one parameter has to be changed, namely power. Sadness needs representation of the object, requiring as a minimal requirement at least dim forms of object constancy. With *disgust* a toxic object is located within the representational field of the subject, be it the body schema or the representational me. The propositional structure is: "You, object, out of me!" (expulsion). The expressive signal, is together with *contempt*, the most frequently used sign of the negative affects in everyday interactions; however, it is rarely mentioned as an introspective mental event. (See Figure 7.1.)

Definition of drives

There are several way to define drives: one approach is for the drives to be defined out of the so-called final acts: that is, we speak of hunger when a person is "driven" to eat, of sexuality when a person is "driven" to genital satisfaction. The defining characteristic is, in Freud's terminology, the handling of the erogenous zones to end their activation. The drive goal [*Triebziel*] would be to end the activation of the drive source [*Triebquelle*], leading to the above-mentioned signal of "*Lust*" as a form of reinforcement.

The other idea considers drives as organizing principles—as, for example, the genital principle. It postulates that these principles themselves are invisible and silent, and that they grow noisy and visible bit by bit only in an affective realization with the partner or the outside world. For both conceptions there are in ethology important considerations:

When we take, for example, the theory of Tinbergen (1966) and Baerends (1956), instincts are to be seen as organizing programmes with the following constants:

- They are hierarchically configured.
- At every hierarchical level there are several antagonistic organizing centres that, once activated, are mutually inhibiting.
- Between the single organizing surfaces there are unspecific behaviour segments, the so-called appetence behaviour.
- The drive cycle ends with the final act, which is the activation of the erogenous zones, leading to discharge experienced as reinforcement (*Lust*).

Running through the whole organization, at every level, it comes to acts, which open up the next type of appetence behaviour: finally the erogenous zones are discharged, leading to the final acts mentioned above, which are identical with the drive concepts—that is, copulating, eating, flight, and so on. Without wanting to transfer the conception of instinct onto human beings, there is enough confirmed knowledge that three hierarchical organized areas with partial antagonisms can be distinguished: the attachment, autonomy, and sexuality motivation systems (Bischof, 1985; Buck, 1976). Although we do not see them as instincts, these systems are in their organizational structure hierarchical and have antagonisms at the same level, a large temporal part being characterized as appetence search behaviour and specific final acts. Given that affects in phylogenesis develop from "appetitive", we will look there for the place they come together (Bischof-Köhler, 1985).

Affects facilitate drive activity when they appear in the same area of organization and inhibit them when they appear in another area.

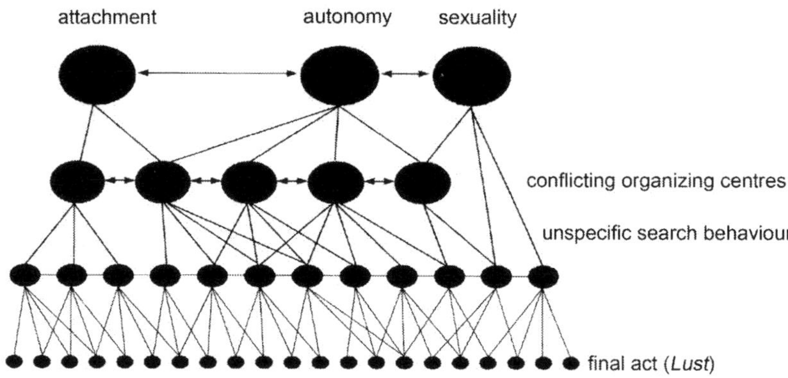

Figure 7.2

Fear, for example, inhibits autonomy and fight but works as a facilitating factor for attachment systems, as shown in the identification-with-the-aggressor phenomenon (Bischof, 1985). Disgust inhibits attachment and incorporation but not autonomy regulation. Happiness facilitates attachment and seduction but inhibits flight and aggression. So usually the first seven months are dominated by happiness encounters—up to 30,000 between mother and child (Emde, 1991). As mentioned above, the affects are embedded in organizing programmes that they fit (Krause, 1991). So the condition for sexual copulation is a general attachment and courtship behaviour—otherwise the partners would not come together. Another condition is that autonomy is more-or-less arranged, otherwise copulation would be settled in a dominance–submission context (Moser, von Zeppelin, & Schneider, 1991).

Reverse linking between affect and drive/motivational organization

Under certain boundary conditions that can end up in pathological solutions, the relation between affect and drive is reversed, and the programme, including the "final act", is used in order to counteract and sedate an affect that seems unbearable. This solution relies on the biological incompatibility of the two. Sadness, for example, is from its propositional structure a call for a lost object that is not yet given up. As long as this phase of the sadness reaction is retained, the "consummatory action" of eating or sexuality does not take place. They are incompatible with the appetence, physiology, and propositional structure of sadness (Krause, 1991). The affect may be reduced by activating the incompatible drive act if eating. Such "consummatory actions" can be used in order to sedate sadness and to keep it from consciousness. The problem is, however, that psychically as well as physiologically drive actions fall under the dominance of the motivation system to be avoided and its affects (Lincke, 1981). Patients become dependent on the drive actions, just because there are no more physiological final criteria, and they have to eat every time they are sad (Krause, 1983). This is the link to addiction that is also typical for perverse behaviour. Inward, the incorporated object acquires the quality of the mourned object that is searched for and has not been given up. Usually the object had been experienced with high ambivalence, which is one of the reasons why it cannot be given up. So the emotional shadow of this object falls on the subject (Freud, 1917e[1915]). This relation is ritually used in the case of "totemism".

Sexual solutions

Anger–Lust, *fear*–Lust

In the case of sexual actions, the affects of fear, anger, and disgust are usually antagonistic to sexual final acts because they are not "appetitive parts "of the attachment and erotic motivation system. Anger belongs as an affect into the area of autonomy regulation. In general it can be stated that anger, with the propositional structure "You, object, go away; I, subject, stay here" cannot be combined with sexual actions because this affect rejects the object. When the anger is not thwarted through something else, it does not come to the approximation of the objects. Under the condition of a subgroup of perversions, which Stoller described as the erotic form of hate, the relation existing between affect and drive is reversed. The appetence anger becomes a necessary precondition for any sexual action. So we have a case of anger–*Lust*. Depending on how severe the pathology is, this can occur in a playful context or it must be acted out as real destruction (Kernberg, 1985, 1991b). The sexual act serves the autonomy regulation and is the guarantee of dominance and power. In the animal kingdom such "*Funktionswechsel*" [change of function] happens very often—for example, in the case of mounting in order to guarantee dominance (Eibl-Eibesfeld, 1984). The same applies to the relation between fear and sexual actions. Under certain conditions the sexual actions are used to sedate and counteract intense feelings of fear. The extremely risky enactments of some perverse acts can be located in this regulatory system. Both affects, anger and fear, and the corresponding motivation conditions change and discharge into sadomasochistic play, where the central point is the fixation in the anal phase for dominance and submission (Novick & Novick, 1991).

Disgust–Lust

Safe attachment is indispensable for a real erotic sexual experience, because empathy for the experience of the other represents the condition for the dissolution of the I/you-limits in orgasm. Normally the affect of disgust totally inhibits this type of motivation systems because it has, as mentioned above, a propositional structure according to which a toxic object that is localized in the self is expelled out of the subject. A very large group of people with very fragile solutions can be characterized by the enactment of sexual relations with an object that would normally provoke massive disgust in the partner. This enactment of disgust now becomes a precondition for the sexual action. One function of the enactment is testing the object whether it can stand the affect without expelling the subject; another is the handling of dangerous fusional ideas between the subject lover and a toxic object that is not supposed to enter the self. This disgust interaction has a restitutive function for the body schema boundaries also, though not for the inner identity. We have pointed out that there is often a compensatory relation between body self and intentional self in such a way that the one can be used to compensate the faulty other (Krause, Steimer-Krause, & Ullrich, 1992). The precarious definition of self-identity is tightened to the body schema, precisely because there are no identity characteristics in the area of the intentional self. All of these patients use external attributes of their body as synonyms with the self. This idolizing of the body and at the simultaneous hollowing out of the intentionality has in fact been described by all authors (Khan, 1979; McDougall, 1986; Morgenthaler, 1984). Against this background the sexual act is one of the rescue fantasies to conserve identity and to inner refill, and the disgust component protects from a diffusion of the I/you-limits during the act. Gallese, Keysers, and Rizzolatti (2004) have shown that seeing and hearing disgust behaviour in others' facial expression or regurgitating activates the same insula regions in experiencing disgust. This means that, at least at the level of the neuroanatomical activation patterns, the I/you boundaries are completely blurred. This has a high survival value. The observing subject learns in one trial that the substance the others were consummating is toxic. Thus the understanding of basic aspects of social cognition depends on the activation of neural structures normally involved in our own personally experienced actions or emotions. In empathy for pain the same structures are activated as those for disgust. The most frequently shown affect in the face on seeing mutilation of a human body is disgust, not fear, and disgust is an affect that is active from birth on—at least in the face of the baby, but also in that of the mother. The problem of which mechanisms mediate the distinction between "who" is really acting and first feeling an emotion when an individual is observing actions is central for the definition of intentionality. On the neuropsychological level some interesting solutions could be found (Jackson & Decety, 2004).

The act of exhibitionism as an example of disgust–*Lust* solution to an identity fissure

The act of exhibitionism is prototypical enactment of a disgust solution:

- Before the initiation of the act, events have taken place that cause the identity, which is in any case very fragile, to almost break into pieces; these events are generally experienced by the patient as a severe offence against self-worth.
- The patient enters into a dissociative state that is in many respects different from his "normal functioning".
- He starts to hunt for subdominant objects (children, women).

- If successful in his search, he suddenly and unexpectedly displays the genitalia, eagerly looking for the affect in the face and voice of his victim.
- If it is disgust and/or fear, the patient can masturbate, and the restitutive act is completed.

The eliciting conditions are not of the nature of the sexual drive but of narcissism—generally identity diffusion elicited through narcissistic injury.

Identity is equated with the sexual identity, which means a narrowing of the self attributes to an idolized body schema.

It results, as described above, in the search for an object that confirms the idolized form of the body schema through specific feedbacks. This can be an affect, pain, usually evoked through aversive acts.

The object is, defined on the basis of its function, a partial object; it is for this reason that non-human objects can also be used as fetishes, and, conversely, human objects can be dehumanized. The person's own image acquires here a prominent role. Looking into the mirror has a magical value for most perverse constructions—either avoiding it at any price during excitement or using it as an intermediate restitutive arrangement that is less dangerous than the real other.

The function of this behaviour is to confirm the existence and functionality of the genitalia, because something that causes spontaneous disgust has to have an existence. After this feedback a kinaesthetic execution in the strict sense of a sexual final act can be materialized. This peak experience with the memory on restitutive behaviours closes the fissures in the identity for a certain time.

Some developmental aspects

The building of the body schema is one of the main pillars of identity formation. The process is tied to the afferent stimuli from the skin and from the inside of the body, but even more so to affects of the caregiver during the handling of the body. The small child perceives the object world along with this his own body according to the affects of "significant others". If the body, and specifically the genital region, are disgusting for the adults, the daily manipulation of this sensory region will be accompanied by facial expressions of disgust. Such expressive dialogues are unconscious and appear very often. In these object relations a Pavlovian conditioning process is put into operation, which results in excitations from this region falling under the dominance of the disgust propositional structure. The drive stimuli are annulled by the affect governing the object relation. It subjectively leads to an extinction of the genital region from the sensory body schema. Phyllis Greenacre had already alluded to this phenomenon in her 1953 paper, "Certain Relationships between Fetishism and Faulty Development of the Body Image". The fetish is a fixed transitional object that has later gained an erotic character, its function being to fill this hole in the sensory body schema. (Greenacre, 1953, 1969; Morgenthaler, 1984). The intense later fear of losing the genitalia (castration anxiety) that is so characteristic for perverse solutions grows on a body schema in which this area of the body already represents a sensory hole.

Structures related to the perverse solutions: psychosis and some eating disorders

There have been numerous attempts to locate perversions in the psychoanalytic nosology. First, a link to psychotic-like processes can be found. Most of these patients have a psychotic lack in the reality perception of the body, especially the genital area (Freud, 1924b). The above-mentioned sensory holes have no external equivalent: the genitalia are there, and they are usually of normal size. The phantasm of having a child's penis can be observed in most cases, especially in paedophiles (Portman, Hale, & Campbell, 2005). The affective erotic misperception of a rubber blanket as an object of desire, as is the case in fetishism, determines at least in this stamped-out area a radically changed reality perception that is under psychotic rule (Rosenfeld, 1984). The reality misperception goes beyond the fetish, however. In a study with sexual offenders who abused children they were in charge of, the most consistent event was that men were convinced that children would have wanted and provoked this kind of "love". Apart from the ignored age difference, the illusive perceptive change in the size of the genitals size has psychotic qualities.

According to our ideas, some eating disorders also show a homology to perverse solutions, which allows us to consider them as part of the perverse structure. The starting point is, as in the case of male perversions, a narcissistic identity disorder. The identity question is fixed to the body schema in a similarly illusive way. To regulate the intolerable affects related to the self a drive action—in this case eating—is used. To expel the toxic object by disgust affects being artificially induced helps to clear the exasperating identity question through the transformation of the body schema. The toxic object was in; now it is out. What is, of course, different is that no open sexual action can be used as terminal reaction for sedation; however, as mentioned above, the nature of "consummatory action" is not constitutive for the problem that is supposed to be resolved.

Some thoughts on treatment techniques

In our study on treatment processes (Merten, 2001), we found a patient with a severe perversion whose disgust pattern was innervated 90 times during the first hour. Although less systematically, I have myself observed a disgust theme in all my patients—through expressive behaviour, clothes, malodour, even to urinating in front of my practice. Now I am working on the profitable hypothesis that these disgust orgies are a mixture of attempts to repair, as described above in the case of exhibitionism, and of a repetition compulsion, though with transposed roles. In the treatment these serve to ensure that the therapist does not feel disgust in face of the patient's person. This occurs in the frame of a "testing-the-limits" proceeding that is activated as long as it is clear, either consciously or unconsciously, that the patient can no longer be contained in his intolerable affects.

I have never been so intensively examined and tested as in the report of perverse actions and facts. The slightest sign of unease is used for destructive fantasies about quitting/abandoning the relation. The patient's transferences oscillate between the fear of a complete rejection, and the apprehension they could include the therapist in their erotized phantoms.

As mentioned earlier, patients very often manage to sail around the perversion theme for quite a long time. One patient related to me after one-and-a-half years of treatment an episode of hunting for boys at the railway station, claiming that this was the last conscious thing that he had deliberately kept secret. In a strange way patients think that we are not "mature" enough for the perversions. If my understanding is correct, maturity refers in the end to the patient's anticipation that we are not able to support and tolerate him in his "being disgusting"/"nastiness". Usually the perverse enactment in treatment is centred around disgust and contempt long before the sexual perversion comes into the open. The patient secretly does more or less disgusting things—including emitting body odours that are very intense—unconsciously governing the countertransference. We should attentively look for and observe these phenomena. They are very often misunderstood as anger or hatred or aggression. This view is not helpful. Their function is to manage closeness of the bodies. There is a very intense countertransference taboo on these affects. To admit disgust is much more difficult than anger because of its antagonistic relation to love and attachment. The patient tests the analyst to see whether he will remain attached to the disgusting subject before he can put the perverse solutions into the discourse. To counteract these tests, it is preferable to empathize with the patient as a child who was a disgusting baby, for example, in mother's nose and eyes. Another constellation I found quite often is that the child's body is idealized—the wonderful bottom, but with the exclusion of the disgusting penis. Starting from this testing function, it is my opinion that patients should, at least at the beginning, be treated in the sitting position, in order to allow them to perceive whether the therapist really feels disgust. It is also easier to elaborate their desperate attempts to abandon the therapy (Krause, 1992). Without this form of reality testing of the countertransference reactions, there is a risk of psychotic breakdowns.

Another facet of the avoidance of talking about the perverse enactment is an intense fear that the magic constructions are so powerful that the analyst will be pulled into the same system, which means that he will not be able to rescue the patient. So not showing the constructions rescues the analyst from getting addicted to the same body magic. There is then an intense fear of losing the magical power of the perverse enactment by talking about it, without having anything else to fill the sensory and intentional holes. So it is not recommended that the patient be forced to abandon it by insisting on working on it before the disgust enactment has come to a satisfying end, with the patient feeling secure that the analyst will remain attached to him after the disclosure. There is strong yet well-hidden enactment of contempt centred around the following themes: "The analyst is too stupid and too weak to find out the secret. . . ." "He has no access to the magic. . . ." "His sexuality is boring. . . ." The strong castration fears make it very difficult for the patient to realize and admit his contempt. It is helpful to admit, at least internally, that the patient has access to things we do not have and that, indeed, we are frequently people to laugh about.

Commentary

Rudi Vermote

When I read Ramachandran's *Phantoms in the Brain* (1998), I had the impression that my scope of understanding unconscious communication was broadened at once. Ramachandran reports the effects of a simple box with a transposing mirror on the perception of phantom limbs. In this mirror-box, the patient's own normal right arm, for example, is seen now at the left side of the body, instead of the phantom limb. The effect is instantaneous and magical: the phantom may relax, become painless, and eventually disappear, even when the patient is aware that the visual effect is an illusion. As a psychoanalyst, I had the impression that this immediate and unconscious reaction to sensory input, without correction by conscious processes at another level of the mind, might explain in part the clinical phenomenon of projective identification.

I discovered later that Rainer Krause (Krause, Steimer-Krause, & Burkhard, 1992) has already been investigating these phenomena of unconscious communication since the 1980s and has developed a psychopathological model of it, with this model relevant to psychosomatic, perverse, hysterical, obsessional, and psychotic structures. Furthermore, Krause developed empirical measures to explore this model: based on his and others' ideas of affects as a evolutionary form of communication, he further developed the FACS (facial action coding system). The FACS (Ekman & Friesen, 1978) descriptively registers each facial movement that is anatomically feasible, based on the innervations of the facial muscles. With this method, he has been able to discern different types of pathology from normal comparisons and has studied non-verbal interactions in psychotherapy between therapist and patient. With his research group at the Saarbrücken University, he identified interaction patterns that distinguished between successful and unsuccessful short psychotherapy treatments.

Today he presents the application of his model to a specific domain: perverse actions, solutions, and structures.

I decided that the best approach was to see whether my clinical practice benefited from the integrative model that Krause presents, taking as my premise that nothing is so practical as a good theoretical model.

We all have, as a kind of toolkit, implicit theories to which we turn in an almost automatic way when at work. With regard to perversion, I rely mainly on the following theories: (1) Kernberg's (1992) distinction of the function and meaning of perverse behaviour according to personality organizations: neurotic, borderline, narcissistic, malignant narcissistic, and antisocial—a distinction that is of enormous clinical value in understanding perverse behaviour; (2) the ideas of Bion (1963) regarding psychic evacuation by action, perverse actions being a way of dealing with unbearable psychic states and the peculiar perverse dynamics of turning the Love, Hate, and Knowledge links into minus Love, minus Hate, and minus Knowledge; (3) the Lacanian notions of the perverse structure (Lacan, 1954) serve, for me, as a kind of warning how one can become relegated to the role of an impotent spectator in the transference–countertransference of patients with a perverse structure, and I also rely on Lacan's description of the dynamics with the law-father and his ideas of the important role of the mother in the aetiology of the perverse structure. I wondered whether I would find these points of reference in Krause's model on perverse behaviour and structure.

Being in charge of a psychoanalytically informed hospital treatment for personality disorders, I often encounter patients displaying so-called "perverse solutions". From experience, we know that when we admit more than one or two such patients at a time, the psychotherapeutic culture of the setting is endangered. Moreover, when the perversion is associated with an antisocial personality organization, it is a contra-indication for the treatment—not so much for the patient but to protect the other patients.

Just before reading Krause's chapter, I had a first interview with a man in his early twenties: he had come to our setting on his own initiative and said that it was his last hope. In a nutshell, he was an only child, pestered at school and accused at age 14 of sexual intimidation towards a 9-year-old girl. He found himself to be the victim of fantasies of this girl. There was further isolation at school, associated with an intense fantasy life full of sexually aggressive phantasies. He failed at his studies and was finally admitted to a psychoanalytic psychotherapeutic centre at 20. During this treatment he was asked to freely associate in group about his inner life. According to his story, he poured out all his sexual phantasies to patients, nurses, and therapists—and everyone was shocked. At the same time, he developed intense feelings of attachment towards a nurse, who felt threatened and stalked by him. He himself denies any stalking activity.

The patient was discharged from this setting as being untreatable, and when he came back to visit this setting, he received a warning that the police would be called if he was seen again in the grounds of the institution. He found this very unfair as, to his mind, he had done what the staff had asked of him—to talk freely about his inner life—but was then punished for it. He told me that he has felt very aggressive internally since, had sexually aggressive fantasies that increased after the rejection, and he was afraid of not being able to control them any more, afraid of becoming verbally and physically aggressive when someone frustrated him.

It struck me that he was telling his story with a mocking smile that made me feel uneasy. Furthermore, nonverbally he appeared arrogant and triumphant, but this seemed at odds with what he reported he was feeling, as his hands were damp with the perspiration of anxiety. I asked him if he was aware of this non-verbal communication, noting that it may set people against him and did not correspond to what he really felt. He said that he was completely unaware of this.

Given his experience in the other centre, it seemed at first unreasonable to admit him. While talking with him, however, it was my impression that he seemed to be aware of an inner suffering, and I had the perhaps naive impression that there was merit to his complaint: that the massive rejection in the other institution had been caused in part by a mechanical application of the psychoanalytic frame with free association and exploration that were not well suited at the given moment to this patient.

In this case, I diagnosed a perverse behaviour in the analytic sense in a patient with malignant narcissism who used a therapeutic setting to evacuate his inner feelings; who used the explicit and vivid wording of his sexual fantasies to project his anxious, oppressed side onto others and control it there; and who was unable to mentalize it or reflect on its impact on others. I was concerned that our setting would become the playground for this as well: we would be reduced to spectators, and in the end would have to stop the treatment prematurely as well. I discussed with the patient that there was a chance that his treatment would fail again. We agreed to offer him a chance under close guidance. The treatment started, and it is, indeed, difficult for the patient to control himself and for the staff to contain the mixture of anxiety and provocative behaviour.

In this treatment Krause's model of impossible combinations in perverse structures is illuminating. We can understand the patient's problem as a combination of the motivational systems of attachment and of seduction with the antagonistic affects of disgust and contempt, affects that he communicates and evokes strongly in a nonverbal way. This understanding makes the peculiar transference–countertransference interactions with this patient more bearable. Staff members can recognize his provocative behaviour as a need for closeness despite evoking affects of disgust and even fear. This is in contrast to interpreting his behaviour as deliberately attacking the setting or abusing the vulnerability of other patients. Understanding the behaviour of the patient as a manifestation of being held hostage by paradoxical patterns, probably stemming from early infancy, is neither judgemental nor moralistic.

Furthermore, Krause's model is not in conflict but adds to our basic points of reference of psychoanalytically informed hospital treatment with a focus on transference, mentalization, and felt safety. Regarding transference, the working through of the impossible combinations has to happen via the working through in the here-and-now of the transference and not by an interpretation of content. Jimenez (2004) discusses this in detail and in relation to Krause's model. With regard to mentalization, it is clear that the perverse solution reflects a failing mentalization: the patient is using the evocation of disgust and a threatening behaviour as a way to regulate his own affects in contact with the therapists and the fellow patients instead of mentalizing them. He has a poor capacity to reflect on what he provokes in others with his behaviour. This results in a misperception of the reality. For instance, he asked a staff member whether he could go with her to the toilet, being sure that she would like this. Within a secure environment it becomes possible to discuss this false perception, to gradually explore his feelings, and look for ways to deal mentally with them

What about the relation of Krause's model to Kernberg's (1992) model of perversion? Here again we see that the two models are not in conflict but enrich each other. Impossible combinations are at the base of all kinds of perverse behaviour—but it makes a difference when this is enacted in reality, as with the presented patient with a low-level borderline personality organization or when it is a playful fantasy, as in patients with a neurotic personality organization.

In conclusion, to me Krause's work is a fine example of how our clinical work can benefit from discoveries and models stemming from psychoanalytic research.

8

Conclusion: future clinical, conceptual, empirical, and interdisciplinary research on sexuality in psychoanalysis

Marianne Leuzinger-Bohleber

> It is to learn, for example, that love and history are related that betrayal of love is conditional upon time that faithfulness and faithlessness depend on the nature of the era in which all of it happens. The respective situation of each historical society strongly affects all procedures of love and betrayal; it influences the structure of feelings and the vitality of passion. Your way of feeling is influenced by particular patterns of the era anyway. The question of how these patterns come about and under which conditions they may alter, basically depends on the accessibility of historical changes to the field of Analysis. . . . [p. 105]
>
> Today, stories about faithlessness, betrayal and vengeance are neither subject of studies dealing with the difference of characters of both sexes—Frailty, thy name is woman; *La donna e mobile*—nor are they pedagogical endeavours to salve civil matrimony and family as it was understood during the nineteenth century. Moreover, these stories are dramatic inquiries coping with the issue of loneliness of moral subjects in Modernity. Law and order are not only missing for betrayal and its retaliation, but also for one's own guilt and the guilt of the others. Characters regard themselves as being murderers, victims and perpetrators, covered by blood just

> like in the ancient tragedy. At the same time they are being tapped on their shoulders by many well-meaning, eloquent understandingly people, saying: live has never been easy for you. . . . [p. 419]
>
> [Peter von Matt, *Liebesverrat*, 1998]

Identity, Gender, and Sexuality: 150 Years after Freud seems a more appropriate title for the publication of the papers presented at the Joseph Sandler Conference, 2005, considering the results and insights of our discussion. The original title of the conference—"Sexual Deviation: 100 years after Freud's *Three Essays on the Theory of Sexuality*"—was due to our common interest in possible changes in psychoanalytic knowledge about what Freud had called "sexual deviation": homosexuality, transsexuality, transvestism, and paedophilia. All the speakers at the conference hinted at the fact that a century after Freud's *Three Essays on the Theory of Sexuality*, we can no longer use the term "sexual deviation". The question of what is "normal" and what is "deviant" in sexuality has become a complex and delicate issue of current psychoanalytic and nonpsychoanalytic discourse that always depends on the societal, cultural, and historical backgrounds in which the question on "normality" arise.

Analysing the extreme transformation in sexuality during recent decades, Sigusch (1998) has created the term "neosexual revolution". In his opinion, its consequences might be even more influential than those of the "sexual revolution" in the 1960s and 1970s. Sexuality has lost its flair as a positive myth, as a realm of liberation, exaltation, and ecstasy. It no longer seems to be the great metaphor for lust and happiness. The "old" sexuality was positively mystified (see, e.g., the influential work of Herbert Marcuse). Nowadays, in contrast, it appears to be negatively mystified: sexuality is associated with inequality of gender, abuse, violence, and deadly infections. During the mystification of "free love", drive, and orgasm, the focus of interest was on the love between heterosexual couples. Neosexuality, by contrast, represents the differences between genders, narcissistic love, thrills and substitute or partial satisfactions. The neosexual revolution is characterized by the media, the commercialization of all forms of sexuality, and the disappearance of intimacy. Sexuality has become a product of the "free market" much more than in former days. Has sexuality—100 years after Freud—thus lost its exclusive function as the most important determining source for psychic development and the longings of human beings? Has the need for attachment, security, and tenderness replaced sexual passion?

The contributors to this book surely agree that *this is a central question to be investigated further,* also by psychoanalysts, although most of them are sceptical with regard to generalizations such as those quoted by Sigusch. But what seems to be beyond any doubt is the fact that sexual relationships have become diversified in such an extreme way that we can hardly speak of "normality" any more. After a long fight for acceptance, in many of the Western countries homosexual couples are allowed to get married and even to adopt children. To change one's sex through surgery has also become possible in these countries. Regarding heterosexuality, we also observe a wide range of diverse forms of sexuality: on the one hand, the number of singles with changing sexual relationships or without sexual practices is increasing; on the other, at least in Germany, the number of constant and stable couples with a new form of fidelity is also on the increase. Adolescents in mass entertainments—such as raves—seem to search for extreme narcissistic autoerotic satisfactions, but at the same time they also looking for romantic love affairs. Therefore all time diagnoses—as, for example, the "Age of Narcissism" (Christopher Lasch), of self-sex (Sigusch) or the exhausted self (Ehrenberg) do not seem to be capable of covering the whole scope of current sexual expressions and relationships.

Such variability and diversity mean an enormous challenge for psychoanalytic theories and clinical practice. Which of Freud's concepts, developed 100 years ago, still offers enough explanatory power to enlighten determinants and manifestations of current sexuality? Which ones have to be modified, or even replaced? These questions all run like red threads through the chapters in this volume.

André Haynal begins chapter two with the central question just mentioned: "Sexuality has been at the centre of interest of psychoanalysis. Is it still today?" André Green (1995) went even further, asking polemically: "Has sexuality anything to do with psychoanalysis?" He has elaborated his observation that sexuality has moved to a marginalized position in psychoanalytic journals as well as in clinical papers and discussions. Is this due to societal changes? Or is Green correct when he postulates that sexuality still plays a central role in the clinical material but would not be recognized by analysts who follow a fashion in psychoanalytic theorizing that concentrates on object relations, pregenital fixations, borderline personality disorders, or early development. As a consequence, sexuality and its role in the psychopathologies would not be recognized precisely enough and would therefore be underestimated. For André Green, a creative survival of psychoanalysis depends essentially on the question of whether genital sexuality and the Oedipus complex will regain their central relevance within psychoanalytic theories. Haynal discusses that it has been Freud himself who—by defining sexuality in a broad way—"opened the door to an advance in such a direction": for an exploration of pregenital pleasure or the narcissistic dimension. Haynal shares Green's position, postulating that "Sex is a powerful organiser of experience" and "Libido is responsible for the bonding between persons . . . Its role in everyday life cannot be exaggerated, creating sympathy, attraction, as well as hostility". Sverre Varvin adds: "Moreover, sex is a powerful organizer of experience, as Haynal also states. Bodily sensations and sensual pleasure define one's skin, and our boundaries and our relation to others are thus formed by the way sexuality shapes fantasies and the structure of the inner world." Therefore, for Haynal, Varvin, and the other contributors to this volume, *regaining the central importance of sexuality in human existence and development guarantees that psychoanalysis does not lose its depth and idiosyncrasy and thus keeps its attraction as a specific discipline of the unconscious for the current interdisciplinary exchange with the scientific community and the public.*

Another red thread running through chapters arising from a *psychoanalytic research conference* is, of course, the question of *how complex clinical and societal phenomena should be adequately researched in psychoanalysis.* In chapter three I give a short overview on a possible interrelationship between clinical, conceptual and empirical research in psychoanalysis, and here I add just a few additional remarks.

Homosexuality

In chapter four, Richard C. Friedman elaborates one danger of *exclusively clinical research in psychoanalysis*: An—unconscious—submission to the ideological views of training analysts may blind one's own eyes to delicate clinical phenomena, like, for example, the homosexuality of patients. "There is no discussing the issue of homosexuality in psychoanalysis without awareness of ideological influences on psychoanalytic thought, political correctness, bias, and prejudice—the latter sometimes denied and acted out." These biases and prejudices of psychoanalytic theorizing on homosexuality have been criticized by political movements—like the "radical gay left"—as well as through discussions in the context of creating the DSM–III by American psychiatrists, who not only criticized the ideological positions on homosexuality in psychoanalysis but also questioned the validity of clinical psychoanalytic research in general. But, as Downey and Friedman (1998) explain, it was not primarily *this kind of psychoanalytic research* that was responsible for the biases but the fact that homosexuality had not been subjected to *careful* clinical studies. The authors were astonished by how undisciplined and chaotic the psychoanalytic literature was and how seldom the knowledge from other scientific disciplines had been taken into account.

Friedman shows that self-critical and sophisticated clinical research in psychoanalysis can be combined in a fruitful way with empirical and interdisciplinary research. A systematic comparison of clinical studies on the treatment of gay patients by psychoanalysts is one of Friedman's basic theoretical foundations for further developing psychoanalytic concepts, comparing and contrasting them with interdisciplinary knowledge from genetics, neurobiology, developmental psychology, and so on. Of course, such new integrations and further theoretical developments are possible only if psychoanalysts "endorse an open-minded, curious, and inquiring attitude towards sexuality".

What can be learned from such an integration of clinical research insights and interdisciplinary knowledge? Gender differences in behaviour are attributable to sexual differentiation of the brain. Prenatal testosterone influences brain embryogenesis. Friedman discusses this biological influence on the different ways boys play compared to how girls play in early, mid-, and late childhood. Systematic studies have shown that homosexuals avoided "rough-and-tumble activities"/RTP) in their early childhood—one factor why they had often been excluded by their peers in latency. "Boys on a gay developmental track are more likely than those on a heterosexual track to be bullied by other boys and men—sometimes including their fathers—because of what I will term here their gender-role temperaments". Friedman postulates that these experiences are much more relevant for the development of homosexuality than oedipal fantasies, as "classical psychoanalysis" has suggested so far. Therefore he postulates that the aggressive components of the oedipal conflict with homosexuals seem to be much more influential than the libidinal ones. These findings are important for clinical practice and should be further studied systematically.

Friedman also discusses the central question whether homosexuals should be "cured" from their homosexuality during a psychoanalytic treatment. Because of his conceptualization of the early (even prenatal) factors influencing a homosexual track of development, he is sceptical. Once sexual fantasies have become part of a stable internally experienced "erotic narrative" during late childhood and adolescence (male masturbation fantasies), they tend to remain more-or-less constant for life. Referring to his clinical experiences, he writes: "Successful treatment, however, seems—at least in my experience—to be associated with a movement away from dehumanized sadistic/masochistic scenarios that are experienced in a rigid and limited way and towards some type of authentic human interaction".

Anne-Marie Sandler—in her commentary on Friedman's chapter—adds to this view: "Although I absolutely agree that psychoanalytic treatment of homosexuals must not aim to alter the patient's sexual orientation, it does seems important to allow them to express and face their internal malaise. Even though today a homosexual is no longer prosecuted or a pariah of society and may possibly marry and even have children, the reality remains that he cannot take part, together with his partner, in the act of reproduction. Sexuality and intercourse may remain exciting and pleasurable, but the experience that intercourse with a loving other can be an act of wondrous creativity is denied to them."

For all these reasons it remains particularly important that heterosexual psychoanalysts are able to reflect on their countertransference fantasies and reactions in order to be able to work productively with homosexual patients.

Thus both intensive clinical and conceptual research are necessary in order to widen our understanding of homosexual patients as well as of the psychodynamics and determinants of homosexuality in general. Particularly female homosexuality still seems to be a "dark continent", even in modern psychoanalysis. In redefining and modifying our psychoanalytic concepts it will be necessary to consider the current (exploding) findings on sexuality in brain research, neurobiology, as well as developmental research. Friedman considers interdisciplinary research as a great chance for future psychoanalytic research also because, as mentioned above, the belief systems of the analysts will be discovered and opened to a critical reflection by such methodologically elaborated and challenging studies.

Transsexualism/transvestism and childhood identity disorder

Friedemann Pfäfflin and Peter Fonagy share their *critical view of single case studies in psychoanalysis*. The most important lesson implicit in chapter six is, however, that "psychoanalytic clinicians do not have the tools or the conceptual framework to integrate experience beyond the single case" (Fonagy). Pfäfflin has seen several hundred transsexual patients, and he illustrates in an impressive way how a variety of different psychodynamics, psychopathologies, and culturally determined wishes and longings might be connected to the impulse to change one's own sex. It is important to know that the majority of transsexual patients are satisfied after having been operated on. But the majority being satisfied does not mean that for any single person surgical operation is the best solution. The former transvestite patient described in chapter three met some transsexual individuals who regretted the operation and—according to his subjective view based on his empathy for their deep disappointment—Mr M stated: "Their fantasy to be able to change sex and gender had turned out to be an illusion. . . . Thus, I think that each transsexual or transvestite patient should go into analysis before the definitive decision to have an operation." Is this due to an idealization of his psychoanalytic treatment, or does he hint at the fact that empirical research, based on a great number of patients, may offer a safer base for making "scientific generalizations" or for gaining an overview of the variety of symptoms, longings, fantasies, as well as affective and cognitive experiences of one's own sexuality? On the other hand, it does not offer us any security in evaluating whether one idiosyncratic person belongs to one category of patients or to the other. Not denying one's own insecurity and "not knowing" but trying to empathize with the individual fate and personality of every new patient seems to remain at the centre of psychoanalytic professionalism. Knowledge gained through empirical or interdisciplinary studies widens the concepts at the back of our minds, our horizon, and may thus help us to reflect self-critically upon the risk of our clinical perception possibly being influenced by prejudices or biases. But it does not offer much help in understanding a specific clinical situation in depth.

Often empirical researchers claim that clinicians—in contrast to (empirical) researchers—need to feel secure in the clinical situation, thus searching for beliefs, even ideologies, and avoiding a self-critical attitude full of doubts. I personally think that this is not true. On the contrary: "good clinicians" share with "good researchers" an attitude of "not knowing", of curiosity, self critique, and a "constant searching for truth" (as opposed to certainty)—and thus an attitude of humility, which Peter Fonagy found so impressive in Friedemann Pfäfflin's chapter.

I wish that he would find a similar attitude in my clinical papers, where I try to rethink the conceptualization of my clinical observations and thus end by doubting and rejecting my former understandings again and again. From my point of view—as I have tried to illustrate—the critical dialogue with my psychoanalytic colleagues as well as interdisciplinary research partners (e.g. those from the field of Embodied Cognitive Science) may have a similar function of triangulation on one's own perceptions, thoughts, and emotions—which may be fruitful for any kind of psychoanalytic research, be it clinical, conceptual, or empirical. I fear that this might not be transparent enough to the reader, because even Linda Mayes, in her excellent discussion, seems to question the value of such clinical papers *per se.* She considers that clinical research has a function only in generating hypotheses that should be tested further in empirical studies. As far as I am concerned, empirical research on clinical observations is just *one* possibility: another one is deepening clinical research, for example by careful and aggregated single case studies contributing to a clinical knowledge base that has a quality different from those of empirical or conceptual research. In my view psychoanalysis—as other scientific disciplines in these times of the "pluralism of sciences"—has developed its own specific research methods, which are suitable to study its specific "research object"—unconscious fantasies and conflicts—as well as its own quality criteria (see, e.g., Leuzinger-Bohleber & Bürgin, 2003; Leuzinger-Bohleber, Fischmann, & Research Committee for Conceptual Research, in press). This is a position of theory of science [*wissenschaftstheoretische Position*] that is discussed controversially in this volume.

In my opinion, Susan Coates offers another excellent example of an *innovative combination of clinical and empirical research* in chapter five, on childhood gender identity disorder. Like Pfäfflin, she has seen a large number of preschool children and thus offers an impressive new view of the development of gender. To mention just one example again: it was new to me that until age 6–7, few children understand that sexual categorization is based on anatomy. Based on this rich clinical experience and many developmental studies, she offers a new view of "normal" gender development in the preschool years. Such empirically based concepts of early development are the background behind the detailed Diagnostic Criteria for Childhood Gender Identity Disorder (CGID), which she describes in detail. She also offers a short overview on epidemiology and hints at the important finding: clinical studies of adolescents with extreme cross-gender behaviour have found a high incidence of peer relation difficulties, depression, and suicidal behaviour.

Equally impressive is the clinical case material of the 5-year-old Colin, who, after two years of treatment, draws his "story". I have never seen such a touching expression of an internalization process of the—pathological—wish of a mother to have a child of the opposite sex to that of the boy. As I described in chapter three, a lack of a capacity on the part of the (depressed) primary object to accept and "love" the gender of the boy has been a common finding in all the clinical case studies of transvestite patients in the psychoanalytic literature that I have found.

As Sheila Spensley points out in her commentary to Coates's chapter, such careful and detailed case material still presents an excellent possibility for what has been called "*case-based learning*" in psychoanalysis. Case narratives inspire other analysts—as Sheila Spensley, in our case—to compare their own clinical experiences with those of our colleagues. We have discussed some of the dangers and difficulties connected to this learning and research culture: but in spite of all the critiques, we should not forget that this kind of communication—in the sense of the *clinical psychoanalytical research* mentioned above—belongs to the best psychoanalysis has to offer! Many cognitive behavioural colleagues have told me that they envied precisely this narrative tradition of psychoanalysis, which has led to such riches of concepts on the psychodynamics, unconscious fantasies and conflicts, traumata, defences, and so forth, of our patients. Therefore we should avoid a denigration of this clinical tradition and, instead, encourage and respect all different kinds of research in psychoanalysis as well as its broad possibility to combine and interrelate their findings!

Although Rainer Krause does not report detailed clinical observations in chapter seven, they are for him, too the starting point for his theoretical elaborations. "One patient was in treatment for his 'depression' for three years without ever mentioning his severe perverse constructions. Seeing me, as his second analyst, he began after a year to talk about bits of these constructions, talking very contemptuously about the lady therapist to whom he had lied all the time without realizing that he was breaking all rules and laws of treatment." The focus of chapter seven lies on the theoretical integration of such clinical findings with a broad knowledge gained in decades of experimental and empirical research in the field of nonverbal communication, affects, and their facial expressions performed by his research team in Zurich and later in Saarbrücken. He also considers interdisciplinary findings, for example, from affect research in the field of academic psychology, ethology, Cognitive Science, and developmental studies. Based on this broad base of knowledge, he develops a new and challenging understanding of perverse actions. To mention just one example of his conceptualizations, Krause shows that under certain conditions that are often called perverse a fixed pattern of antagonistic coupling of affect and terminal acts is developed, leading to situations whereby sexual lust is linked to affects like fear and disgust. He considers that the drive action is used to sedate the unbearable affect. The developmental origins of such patterns are discussed, with disgust reactions on the side of the caregiver leading to faulty body schema developments in the realm of the genital area. The perverse sexual actions with the object are attempts to re-establish a non-psychotic sensory representational schema.

Therefore Krause's chapter might serve as an example of what we have called *integrative conceptual research* developing further and even re-thinking, re-creating, and developing further central psychoanalytic concepts such as "drive", "affect", and "perverse actions". In spite of all the empirical and interdisciplinary findings that Krause considers, his integrative theorizing remains speculative in the best sense of the word: thinking is still the heart of any science! Of course this is particularly true for a science of the unconscious, psychoanalysis. *Future research in psychoanalysis will thus depend to a great part on such creative and innovative thinkers and theoreticians taking up new clinical and extraclinical observations and integrating them into new and potent psychoanalytic concepts.*

Summary

All the contributors to this volume agree that understanding sexuality in its current manifestations, its "normalities" and "pathologies", its relevance to illness and the process of recovery from trauma and failed developments within the therapeutic dyad and other relationships remains a central topic for future psychoanalytic research. Sexuality has to be rediscovered by psychoanalysis as its genuine field of research, which earns a high priority in our everyday clinical practice as well as in theorizing and research. Some disagreement does exist between the authors of these chapters in their evaluations of which research pathways seem the most promising for psychoanalysis in order to contribute to enlarging the scientific knowledge base on such a delicate, divergent, multidimensional, and biologically as well as socially determined field. Peter Fonagy, for example, sees the main future opportunities in empirical infant research. "In my view . . . *observations of infant development will provide the long-awaited model of human sexuality that psychoanalysis has missed since its inception.*" Others prefer different combinations of clinical, conceptual, and empirical research integrating clinical psychoanalytical and extraclinical (interdisciplinary) knowledge. For some, clinical psychoanalytical investigations should not be seen as a specific form of research, in contrast to the position of others, for whom psychoanalysis, as a clinical science of the unconscious, still seems indispensable in order to investigate the complex field of human sexuality that is always connected with the darkest, most dangerous, but at the same time the brightest and most touching sides of the human existence.

Thus sexuality and love—PSYCHE and AMOR—constitute an inseparable couple, an insight psychoanalysis shares with philosophers, artists, and writers (see the epigraph by Peter von Matt at the beginning of this chapter). To remind us of the innumerable impressive examples in world literature, I would therefore like to close by quoting Anne Michaels *Fugitive Pieces:*

The 7-year-old Jakob Beer is saved by the Greek archaeologist Athos in Poland during the Second World War. Athos smuggles the starving little boy, who has seen his parents murdered by the Nazis and who could not find his little sister either, to Greece and helps him to survive there. His empathy and sensitivity enable him finally to gain the trust of the severely traumatized Jakob. But only in Canada, as an adult man, does Jakob—loved by Michaela—partially become capable to mourn and to re-find himself.

> I'd never heard of you until, in class, Salman recommended your book of poems, *Groundwork*, and recited the opening lines. Later I saw that the book was dedicated to the memory of your parents and your sister, Bella. My love for my family has grown for years in decay-fed soil, an unwashed root pulled suddenly from the ground. Bulbous as a beet, a huge eye under a lid of earth. Scoop out the eye, blind the earth. . . .
>
> In your later poems, it's as if history reads over our shoulder. . . . One couldn't help but feel the force of your presence, your heavy hand as a cat on Michaela's thigh. What is love at first sight but the response of a soul crying out with sudden regret because it realizes it has never before been recognized? [Michaels, 1996, pp. 206, 207]

REFERENCES AND BIBLIOGRAPHY

** Entries with an asterisk represent additional important sources not cited in the text.*

Abraham, N., & Torok, M. (1984). "The lost object—me": Note on identification within the crypt. *Psychoanalytic Inquiry, 4*: 221–242.

American Psychiatric Association (1980). *Diagnostic and Statistical Manual of Mental Disorders* (3rd edition). Washington, DC: American Psychiatric Press.

American Psychiatric Association (1992). *Proposal for Diagnostic and Statistical Manual of Mental Disorders* (4th edition). Washington, DC: American Psychiatric Press.

Baerends, G. P. (1956). Aufbau tierischen Verhaltens. In: W. Kükental (Ed.), *Handbuch der Zoologie, Vol. 8* (pp. 1–32). Berlin: De Gruyter.

Bailey, J. M., & Benishay, D. (1993). Familial aggregations of female sexual orientation. *American Journal of Psychiatry, 150*: 272–277.

Bailey, J. M., Dunne, M. P., & Martin, N. G. (2000). Genetic and environmental influences on sexual orientation and its correlates in an Australian twin sample. *Journal of Personality and Social Psychology, 78*: 524–536.

Bailey, J. M., & Pillard, R. C. (1991). A genetic study of male sexual orientation. *Archives of General Psychiatry, 48*: 1089–1097.

Bailey, J. M., Pillard, R. C., Neale, M. C., & Argei, Y. (1993). Heritable factors influence sexual orientation in women. *Archives of General Psychiatry, 50*: 217–223.

Bailey, J. M., & Zucker, K. J. (1995). Childhood sex-typed behavior and sexual orientation: A conceptual analysis and quantitative review. *Developmental Psychology, 31*: 43–55.

*Bak, R. (1968). The phallic woman: The ubiquitous fantasy in perversion. *Psychoanalytic Study of the Child, 23*: 15–36.

*Bak, R., & Stewart, W. (1974). Fetishism, transvestism and voyeurism: A psychoanalytic approach. In: *American Handbook of Psychiatry, III* (2nd edition, pp. 352–363). New York: Basic Books.

Balint, M. (1965). *Primary Love and Psycho-Analytic Technique.* London: Tavistock.

Baumeister, R. F. (2000). Gender differences in erotic plasticity: The female sex drive as socially flexible and responsive. *Psychological Bulletin, 126* (3): 375–380.

Bayer, R. V. (1981). *Homosexuality and American Psychiatry: The Politics of Diagnosis.* New York: Basic Books.

*Beigl, H., & Feldman, R. (1963). The male transvestite in fiction, research and reality. In: H. Beigl (Ed.), *Advances in Sex Research* (pp. 198–210). New York: Norton.

Bem, S. L. (1989). Genital knowledge and gender constancy in preschool children. *Child Development, 60*: 649–662.

Benjamin, H. (1966). *The Transsexual Phenomenon.* New York: Julian Press.

Bennett, A. (1968). *40 Years On.* London: Faber & Faber.

Bieber, I., Dain, H. J., Dince, P. R., Drellich, M. G., Grand, H. G., Gundlach, R. H., Kremer, M. W., Rifkin, A. H., Wilbur, C. B., & Bieber, T. B. (1962). *Homosexuality: A Psychoanalytic Study of Male Homosexuals.* New York: Basic Books.

Bion, W. R. (1962). *Learning from Experience.* New York: Jason Aronson.

Bion, W. R. (1963). *Elements of Psycho-Analysis.* New York: Jason Aronson, 1977.

Bion, W. R. (1965). *Transformations.* London: Heinemann.

Birkenfeld-Adams, A., Zucker, K. J., & Bradley, S. J. (1998). "Boys with gender identity disorder: Signs of separation anxiety and distress." Poster presented at the Second International Conference on Attachment and Psychopathology, Toronto, Ontario.

Bischof, N. (1989). Emotionale Verwirrungen (Oder: Von den Schwierigkeiten im Umgang mit der Biologie). *Psychologische Rundschau, 40*: 188–205.

Bischof, N. (1985). *Das Rätsel Ödipus.* Munich: Piper.

Bischof-Köhler, D. (1985). Zur Physiologie menschlicher Motivationen. In: L. H. Eckensberger & E. Lantermann (Ed.), *Emotionalität und Reflexivität.* Munich: Urban & Schwarzenberg.

*Blos, P. (1979). *The Adolescent Passage.* New York: International Universities Press.

Blumer, H. (1969). *Symbolic Interactionism: Perspective and Method.* Englewood Cliffs, NJ: Prentice-Hall.

Bohleber, W. (1982). Spätadoleszente Entwicklungsprozesse. Ihre Bedeutung für Diagnostik und psychotherapeutische Behandlung von Studenten. In: E. Krejci & W. Bohleber (Eds.), *Spätadoleszente Konflikte* (pp. 52–81). Göttingen: Vandenhoeck u. Ruprecht.

Bohleber, W. (2000). Die Entwicklung der Traumatheorie in der Psychoanalyse. *Psyche, 54*: 797–839.

*Borsig, B., Rodewig, K., & Wiodera, R. (1993). Die Klassifikation von Sexualstörungen in der ICD–10. In: W. Schneider, H. J. Freyberger, A. Muhs, & G. Schüßler (Eds.), *Diagnostik und Klassifikatioon nach ICD–10, Kap. V* (pp. 200–209). Göttingen: Vandenhoeck u. Ruprecht.

Boss, M. (1950–51). "Erwiderung zum Bericht über mein Referat." Sixty-sixth Peripatetic Meeting of South-West German Psychiatrists and Neurologists, Badenweiler, 2–3 June. *Psyche, 4*: 394–400.

Bradley, S. (1985). Gender disorders in childhood: A formulation. In: B. W. Steiner (Ed.), *Gender Dysphoria: Development, Research, Management* (pp. 175–188). New York: Plenum Press.

Bradley, S. (1990). Affect regulation and psychopathology: Bridging the mind–body gap. *Canadian Journal of Psychiatry, 35*: 540–546.

Bradley, S. J. (2000). *Affect Regulation and the Development of Psychopathology.* New York: Guilford Press.

Bradley, S. J., Zucker, K. J., Gladding, J., et al. (1984). "Gender-dysphoric adolescents: Presenting and developmental characteristics." Paper presented at the joint meeting of the American Academy of Child Psychiatry and the Canadian Academy of Child Psychiatry, Toronto, Ontario, Canada (October).

Braun-Scharm, H., & Loeben-Sprengel, S. (1988). Einige Aspekte der Psychotherapie mit transsexuellen Jugendlichen. *Praxis der Psychotherapie und Psychosomatik, 33*: 258–267.

Breedlove, S. M. (1994). Sexual differentiation of the human nervous system. *Annual Review of Psychology, 45*: 389–418.

Britton, R., Feldman, M., & O'Shaughnessy, E. (1989). *The Oedipus Complex Today: Clinical Implications.* London: Karnac.

Buck, R. (1976). *Human Motivation and Emotion.* New York: Wiley.

Budd, S. (2001). "No sex, please: we're British": Sexuality in English and French psychoanalysis. In: C. Harding (Ed.), *Sexuality: Psychoanalytic Perspectives* (pp. 52–68). Hove: Brunner-Routledge.

*Bürger-Prinz, H., Albrecht, H., & Giese, H. (1953). *Zur Phänomenologie des Transvestitismus bei Männern.* Stuttgart: Enke.

Burzig, G. (1982). Der Psychoanalytiker und der transsexuelle Patient. Ein Beitrag zur notwendigen Auseinandersetzung mit "psycho"-chirurgischen Eingriffen an den Geschlechtsmerkmalen. *Psyche, 36*: 848–856.

Busch de Ahumada, L. C. (2003). Clinical notes on a case of transvestism in a child. *International Journal of Psychoanalysis, 84*: 291–313.

Calogeras, R. C. (1987). The transvestite and his wife. *Psychoanalytic Review, 74*: 517–535.

Cauldwell, D. C. (1949). Psychopathia transsexualis. *Sexology, 16*: 274–280.

Chasseguet-Smirgel, J. (1980). "Réflexions sur la perte de la réalité dans la perversion (avec référence particulière au fetichisme)." Unpublished lecture, SGP, Zurich (19 September).

Chasseguet-Smirgel, J. (1983). Perversion and the universal law. *International Review of Psychoanalysis, 10*: 293–301.

Chasseguet-Smirgel, J. (1985). *Creativity and Perversion.* London: Free Association Books. [*Kreativität und Perversion.* Frankfurt a.M.: Nexus, 1986.]

Chiland, C. (1988). Das geschlechtliche Schicksal des Menschen. In: J. Stork (Ed.), *Das menschliche Schicksal zwischen Individuation und Identifizierung* (pp. 133–153). Stuttgart: Frommann-Holzboog.

*Chiland, C. (1997). *Changes de sexe.* Paris: Odile Jacob.

*Chiland, C. (1998). Panel: Transvestism and transsexualism. *International Journal of Psychoanalysis, 79*: 156–159.

Chiland, C. (2000). The psychoanalyst and the transsexual patient. *International Journal of Psychoanalysis, 81*: 21–35.

Chiland, C. (2003). *Le transsexualisme.* Paris: Presses Universitaires de France.

Chodorow, N. (1994). *Femininities, Masculinities, Sexualities: Freud and Beyond.* London: Free Association Books.

*Chodorow, N. J. (1995). On a case of transsexualism by R. Stein. *Psychoanalytic Dialogues, 5*: 291–300.

Clancey, W. J. (1991). The frame of reference problem in the design of intelligent machines. In: K. van Lehn (Ed.), *Architecture of Intelligence.* Hillsdale, NJ: Lawrence Erlbaum.

*Coates, S. (1990). Ontogenesis of boyhood gender identity disorder. *Journal of the American Academy of Psychoanalysis, 18*: 414–438.

Coates, S. (2005). "Childhood gender identity disorder and the Book of Names." Presented at the American Psychological Association, Division 39.

Coates, S., Friedman, R., & Wolfe, S. (1991). The etiology of boyhood gender identity disorder: A model for integrating psychodynamics, temperament and development. *Psychoanalytic Dialogues, 1*: 481–523.

Coates, S. W., Hahn-Burke, S., & Wolfe, S. (1994). "Do boys with gender identity disorder have a shy, inhibited temperament?" Paper presented at the International Academy for Sex Research, Edinburgh (June).

Coates, S. W., Hahn-Burke, S., Wolfe, S., Shindledecker, R., & Nierenberger, O. (1994). "Sensory reactivity in boys with gender identity disorder: A comparison with matched controls." Paper presented at the International Academy for Sex Research, Edinburgh (June).

Coates, S. W., & Moore, M. S. (1997). The complexity of early trauma: Representation and transformation. *Psychoanal. Inq., 17*: 286–311.

Coates, S., & Person, E. S. (1985). Extreme boyhood femininity: Isolated finding or pervasive disorder? *Journal of the American Academy of Child Psychiatry, 24*: 702–709.

Coates, S. W., & Wolfe, S. (1995). Gender identity disorder in boys: The interface of constitution and early experience. *Psychoanalytic Inquiry, 15*: 6–38.

Coates, S. W., & Wolfe, S. M. (1997). Childhood gender identity disorder. In: A. F. Lieberman, S. Wieder, & E. Fenichel (Eds.), *The DC: 0–3 Casebook.* Washington, DC: Zero to Three.

Cohen-Kettenis, P., & Pfäfflin, F. (2003). *Transgenderism and Intersexuality in Childhood and Adolescence: Making Choices.* Thousand Oaks, CA: Sage.

Coltart, N. E. (1985). The treatment of a transvestite. *Psychoanalytic Psychotherapy, 1*: 65–79.

Cook, C. (1999). "Paternal contributions to the etiology of gender identity disorder: A study of attachment, affect regulation and gender conflict." PhD dissertation, City University of New York.

Cooper, A. M. (1991). "Evaluation of the 37th IPA Congress." Final overview panel, Thirty-Seventh Congress of the International Psychoanalytical Association, Buenos Aires.

Cooper, A. M., Kernberg, O. F., & Person, E. S. (Eds.) (1989). *Toward the Second Century.* New Haven, CT: Yale University Press.

Damasio, A. R. (1994). *Descartes' Error.* New York: Putnam.

de Marneffe, D. (1997). Bodies and words: A study of gender in early childhood. *Gender and Psychoanalysis, 2*: 3–33.

Désirat, K. (1985). *Die transsexuelle Frau.* Stuttgart: Enke.

Diamond, M. (1982). Sexual identity, monozygotic twins reared in discordant sex roles and a BBC follow-up. *Archives of Sexual Behavior, 11*: 181–186.

Diamond, M. (1997). Sexual identity and sexual orientation in children with traumatized or ambiguous genitalia. *Journal of Sex Research, 34*: 199–211.

Diamond, M., & Sigmundson, K. (1997). Sex reassignment of birth: Long-term review and clinical implications. *Archives of Pediatric and Adolescent Medicine, 151*: 298–303.

DiCeglie, D., & Freedman, D. (Eds.) (1998). *A Stranger in My Own Body: Atypical Gender Identity Development and Mental Health.* London: Karnac.

Domenici, T., & Lesser, R. C. (1995). *Disorienting Sexuality: Psychoanalytic Reappraisals of Sexuality Identities.* New York: Routledge.

Dowling, S. (Ed.) (1989). *The Significance of Infant Observational Research for Clinical Work with Children, Adolescents, and Adults.* Madison, CT: International Universities Press.

Downey, J. I., & Friedman, R. C. (1998). Female homosexuality: Classical psychoanalytic theory reconsidered. *Journal of the American Psychoanalytic Association, 46*: 471–506.

Drescher, J. (1998). *Psychoanalytic Therapy and the Gay Man.* Hillsdale, NJ: Analytic Press.

Duberman, M. (1991). *Cures: A Gay Man's Odyssey.* New York: Dutton.

Eckert, E. D., Bouchard, J., Bohlen, J., & Heston, L. (1986). Homosexuality in monozygotic twins raised apart. *British Journal of Psychiatry, 148*: 421–425.

Edelman, G. M. (1987). *Neural Darwinism.* New York: Basic Books.

*Edelman, G. M. (1989). *The Remembered Present: A Biological Theory of Consciousness.* New York: Basic Books.

Edelman, G. M. (1992). *Bright Air, Brilliant Fire.* New York: Basic Books.

Ehrenberg, D. (1993). *The Intimate Edge.* New York: Norton.

Ehrhardt, A. A., & Meyer-Bahlburg, H. F. L. (1981). Effects of prenatal sex hormones on gender-related behavior. *Science, 211*: 1312–1318.

Eibl-Eibesfeld, I. (1984). *Die Biologie des menschlichen Verhaltens.* Munich: Piper.

*Eicher, W. (1984). *Transsexualismus.* Stuttgart, Jena, New York: G. Fischer.

Ekins, R. (1997). *Male Femaling: A Grounded Theory Approach to Cross-Dressing and Sex-Changing.* London/New York: Routledge.

Ekins, R., & King, D. (1996). *Blending Genders: Social Aspects of Cross-Dressing and Sex-Changing*. London, New York: Routledge.

Ekins, R., & King, D. (2006). *The Transgender Phenomenon*. Thousand Oaks, CA: Sage.

Ekman, P., & Friesen, W. V. (1978). *Manual for the Facial Action Coding System*. Palo Alto, CA: Consulting Psychologist's Press.

Emch, M. (1944). On the "need to know" as related to identification and acting out. *International Journal of Psychoanalysis, 25*: 13–19.

Emde, R. N. (1980). Emotional availability: A reciprocal reward system for infants and parents with implications for prevention of psychosocial disorders. In: P. M. Taylor (Ed.), *Parent–Infant Relationships* (pp. 87–115). Orlando, FL: Grune & Stratton.

Emde, R. N. (1983). The prerepresentational self and its affective core. *Psychoanalytic Study of the Child, 38*: 165–192.

Emde, R. N. (1991). Positive emotions for psychoanalytic theory: Surprises from infancy research and new directions. *Journal of the American Psychoanalytical Association, 39*: 5–44.

Emde, R. N. (1992). Positive emotions for psychoanalytic theory: Surprises from infancy research. New directions. In: T. Shapiro & R. N. Emde (Eds.), *Affect: Psychoanalytic Perspectives* (pp. 5–44). Madison, CT: International Universities Press.

Endres de Oliveira, G., & Krause, R. (1989). Reagieren Kleinkinder auf affektive mimische Reize affektiv? *Acta Paedopsychiatrica, 52*: 26–35.

Erikson, E. H. (1950). *Childhood and Society*. New York: Norton.

Erikson, E. H. (1968). *Youth and Crisis*. New York: Norton.

Eshel, O. (2005). Pentheus rather than Oedipus: On perversion, survival and analytic "presencing". *International Journal of Psychoanalysis, 86*: 1071–1099.

Fagot, B. I. (1985). Changes in thinking about early sex role development. *Developmental Review, 5*: 83–98.

Fagot, B. I. (1993). *Gender Role Development in Early Childhood: Environmental Input, Internal Construction*. Pacific Grove, CA: International Academy of Sex Research.

Fairbairn, R. (1952). *Psycho-Analytic Studies of the Personality*. London: Tavistock.

Fast, I. (1984). *Gender Identity: A Differentiation Model*. Hillsdale, NJ: Analytic Press. [German edition: *Von der Einheit zur Differenz*. Berlin/Heidelberg/New York: Springer, 1991.]

Feldman, M. (1999). Projektive Identifizierung. *Psyche-Z. Psychoanal., 53*: 991–1014.

Fenichel, O. (1930). Zur Psychologie des Transvestitismus. *Internazionale Zeitschrift der Psychoanalyse, 16*: 21–34.

Fine, G. A. (1987). *With the Boys: Little League Baseball and Preadolescent Culture*. Chicago, IL: University of Chicago Press.

*Fisk, N. (1973). Gender dysphoria syndrome: The how, what, and why of a disease. In: D. Laub & P. Gandy (Eds.), *Proceedings of the Second Interdisci-*

plinary Symposium on Gender Dysphoria Syndrome (pp. 7–14). Stanford, CA: University of California Press.

Fletcher, J. (1992). The letter in the unconscious: The enigmatic signifier in the work of Jean Laplanche. In: J. Fletcher & M. Stanton (Eds.), *Jean Laplanche: Seduction, Translations, Drives* (pp. 93–120). London: Institute of Contemporary Arts.

Fliess, W. (1897). *Die Beziehungen zwischen Nase und weiblichen Geschlechtsorganen: In ihrer biologischen Bedeutung dargestellt.* Leipzig/Vienna: Franz Deuticke.

Fogel, G. I., & Myers, W. A. (Eds.) (1991). *Perversions and Near-Perversions: New Psychoanalytic Perspectives.* New Haven, CT/London: Yale University Press.

Fonagy, P. (2001). Infantile sexuality as creative process. *Infantile Attachment and Sexuality* (pp. 55–64), ed. D. Widlöcher. New York: Other Press.

Fonagy, P. (2005). "Attachment, trauma and psychoanalysis: Where psychoanalysis meets neuroscience." Unpublished keynote lecture, Forty-Fourth IPA Congress on Trauma, Rio de Janeiro.

Fonagy, P., Gergely, G., Jurist, E. L., & Target, M. (2002). *Affect Regulation, Mentalization, and the Development of the Self.* New York: Other Press.

Fonagy, P., & Target, M. (1997). Perspectives on the recovered memories debate. In: J. Sandler & P. Fonagy (Eds.), *Recovered Memories of Abuse: True or False?* (pp. 183–217). London: Karnac.

Fonagy, P., & Target, M. (submitted). Getting sex back into psychoanalysis.

Francesconi, H. (1984). Transvestitismus beim Mann. *Psyche, 38*: 800–816.

Freud, E. L. (Ed.) (1960). *Letters of Sigmund Freud.* New York: Basic Books.

Freud, S. (1900a). *The Interpretation of Dreams. SE, 4–5.*

Freud, S. (1905d). *Three Essays on the Theory of Sexuality. SE, 7* (pp. 123–243).

Freud, S. (1908c). On the sexual theories of children. *SE, 9.*

Freud, S. (1910c). *Leonardo da Vinci and a Memory of His Childhood. SE, 11.*

Freud, S. (1912f). Contribution to a discussion on masturbation. *SE, 12* (pp. 243–254).

*Freud, S. (1914c). On narcissism: An introduction. *SE, 14.*

Freud, S. (1915c). Instincts and their vicissitudes. *SE, 14.* [Triebe und Triebschicksale. *GW, 10* (pp. 210–232).]

Freud, S. (1916–17). *Introductory Lectures on Psycho-Analysis. SE, 16.*

Freud, S. (1917e[1915]). Mourning and melancholia. *SE, 14.*

Freud, S. (1919e). A child is being beaten. *SE, 17.*

Freud, S. (1920a). The psychogenesis of a case of homosexuality. *SE, 18.*

Freud, S. (1920g). *Beyond the Pleasure Principle. SE, 18.*

Freud, S. (1923b). *The Ego and the Id. SE, 19* (pp. 12–66).

Freud, S. (1924b). Neurosis and psychosis. *SE, 19.* [Der Realitätsverlust bei Neurose und Psychose. *GW, 13* (pp. 360–368). Neurose und Psychose. *GW, 13* (pp. 387–391).]

Freud, S. (1924c). The economic problem of masochism. *SE, 19.*

Freud, S. (1924d). The dissolution of the Oedipus complex. *SE, 19* (pp. 173–182).

Freud, S. (1925j). Some psychical consequences of the anatomical distinction between the sexes. *SE, 19.*

Freud, S. (1927a). Postscript to the question of lay analysis. *SE, 20.*

Freud, S. (1927e). Fetishism. *SE, 21.*

Freud, S. (1931b). Female sexuality. *SE, 21.*

Freud, S. (1933a). *New Introductory Lectures on Psycho-Analysis. SE, 22.*

Freud, S., & Fliess, W. (1985). *The Complete Letters of Sigmund Freud to Wilhelm Fliess, 1887–1904.* Cambridge, MA: Harvard University Press.

Friedman, R. C. (1988). *Male Homosexuality: A Contemporary Psychoanalytic Perspective.* New Haven, CT: Yale University Press.

Friedman, R. C. (1998). Gender identity. *Psychiatric News, 33* (2): 10–31.

Friedman, R. C., & Downey, J. (1994). Special article: Homosexuality. *New England Journal of Medicine, 331*: 923–930.

Friedman, R. C., & Downey, J. (1995a). Biology and the oedipus complex. *Psychoanalytic Quarterly, 54*: 234–264.

Friedman, R. C., & Downey, J. (1995b). Internalized homophobia and the negative therapeutic reaction in homosexual men. *Journal of the American Academy of Psychoanalysis, 23*: 99–113.

Friedman, R. C., & Downey, J. (2002). *Sexual Orientation and Psychoanalysis: Sexual Science and Clinical Practice.* New York: Columbia University Press.

Friedman, R. C., & Downey, J. (2004). On homosexuality: Coming out of the confusion. *International Journal of Psychoanalysis, 85*: 521–523.

Friedman, R. C., Green, R., & Spitzer, R. (1976). Reassessment of homosexuality and transsexualism. *Annual Review of Medicine, 27*: 57–62.

Friedman, R. C., Richart, R. M., & Vande Wiele, R. L. (Eds.) (1974). *Sex Differences in Behavior.* New York: Wiley.

Friedman, R. C., Wollesen, F., & Tendler, R. (1976). Psychological development and blood levels of sex steroids in male identical twins of divergent sexual orientation. *Journal of Nervous and Mental Disease, 163* (4): 282–288.

*Gabbard, G. O. (1991). Technical approaches to transference hate in the analysis of borderline patients. *International Journal of Psychoanalysis, 72*: 625–637.

Gallese, V., Keysers, C., & Rizzolatti, G. (2004). A unifying view of the basis of social cognition. *Trends in Cognitive Sciences, 8*: 396–403.

*Garber, M. (1992). *Vested Interests—Cross-Dressing and Cultural Anxiety.* New York: Routledge.

*Garfinkel, H. (1967). *Studies in Ethnomethodology.* Englewood Cliffs, NJ: Prentice-Hall.

*Garfinkel, H. (1987). *The Sissy Boy Syndrome and the Development of Homosexuality.* New Haven, CT/London: Yale University Press.

George, C., Kaplan, N., & Main, M. (1985). "The Berkeley Adult Attachment Interview." Unpublished protocol, Department of Psychology, University of California, Berkeley.

Gergely, G., & Watson, J. (1996). The social biofeedback model of parental affect-mirroring. *International Journal of Psychoanalysis, 77*: 1181–1212.

*Gershman, H. (1970). The role of core gender identity in the genesis of Perversion. *American Journal of Psychoanalysis, 30*: 58–67.

Gerzi, S. (2005). Trauma, narcissism and the two attractors in trauma. *International Journal of Psychoanalysis, 86*: 1033–1051.

Gibson, L. (1998). "Adult attachment and maternal representations of gender during pregnancy: Their impact on the child's subsequent gender-role development." PhD dissertation, City University of New York.

Giddens, A. (1992). *The Transformation of Intimacy: Sexuality, Love and Eroticism in Modern Societies.* Cambridge: Polity Press.

*Gillespie, W. H. (1952). Notes in the analysis of sexual perversions. *International Journal of Psychoanalysis, 33*: 397–402.

GIRES (2004). *Gender Dysphoria* (flyer, August). Ashtead: GIRES.

Glass, L. L. (2003). The gray areas of boundary crossings and violations. *American Journal of Psychotherapy, 57* (4): 429–444.

Glasser, M. (1992). The management of perversions, with special reference to transvestism. In: R. Lincoln (Ed.), *Psychosexual Medicine.* London: Chapman & Hall.

Glasser, M. (1979). Some aspects of the role of aggression in the perversion. In: I. Rosen (Ed.), *Sexual Deviation* (pp. 278–306). New York: Oxford University Press.

Goldberg, A. (1995). *The Problem of Perversion: The View from Self Psychology.* New Haven, CT/London: Yale University Press.

*Golosow, N., & Weitzman, E. L. (1969). Psychosexual and ego regression in the male transsexual. *Journal of Nervous and Mental Disease, 4*: 328–336.

Gorski, R. A. (1991). Sexual differentiation of the endocrine brain and its control. In: M. Motta (Ed.), *Brain Endocrinology* (2nd edition, pp. 71–103). New York: Raven.

Grand, S. (1997). On the gendering of traumatic dissociation. A case of mother–son incest. *Gender and Psychoanalysis, 2*: 55–77.

Green, A. (1986). The dead mother. In: *On Private Madness* (pp. 142–173). Madison, CT: International Universities Press.

Green, A. (1995). Has sexuality anything to do with psychoanalysis? *International Journal of Psychoanalysis, 76*: 871–883.

Green, A. (1997a). *Les chaînes d'Eros. Actualité.* Paris: Odile Jacob.

Green, A. (1997b). Opening remarks to a discussion of sexuality in contemporary psychoanalysis. *International Journal of Psychoanalysis, 78*, 345–350.

Green, A. (1999). The greening of psychoanalysis. André Green in dialogues with Cregorio Kohon. In: G. Kohon (Ed.), *The Dead Mother.* London: Routledge, 10–58.

*Green, R. (1974). *Sexual Identity Conflict in Children and Adults.* New York: Basic Books.

*Green, R. (1987a). Gender identity in childhood and later sexual orientation: Follow-up of 78 males. *Americal Journal of Psychiatry, 142*: 339–341.

Green, R. (1987b). *The "Sissy Boy Syndrome" and the Development of Homosexuality.* New Haven, CT: Yale University Press.

Greenacre, P. (1953). Certain relationships between fetishism and faulty development of the body image. *Psychoanalytic Study of the Child, 8*: 79–98.

Greenacre, P. (1969). The fetish and transitional object. *Psychoanalytic Study of the Child, 24*: 144–164.

Greenson, R. R. (1966). A transvestite boy and a hypothesis. *International Journal of Psychoanalysis, 47*: 396–403.

*Greenson, R. R. (1968). Dis-identifying from mother. Its special importance for the boy. *International Journal of Psychoanalysis, 49*: 370–374. [German: Die Beendigung der Identifizierung mit der Mutter und ihre besondere bedeutung für den Jungen. In: *Psychoanalytische Erkundungen* (pp. 257–264). Stuttgart: Klett Cotta, 1982.]

Grunberger, B. (1971). *Le narcissisme.* Paris: Payot.

Gutheil, T. G., & Gabbard, G. O. (1993). The concept of boundaries in clinical practice: Theoretical and risk-management dimensions. *American Journal of Psychiatry*, 150 (2): 188–196.

Gutowski, J. S. (2000). A boy who was a girl . . . *Modern Psychoanalysis, 25*: 191–197.

Habel, H. (1950). Zwillingsuntersuchungen an Homosexuellen. *Zeitschrift für Sexualforschung, 1*: 161–180.

Hahn-Burke, S.(1998). "Gender identity disorder, maternal attachment and reflective functioning." PhD dissertation, Ferkauf Graduate School of Psychology, Yeshiva University.

Hamer, D. H., Hu, S., Magnuson, V. L., Hu, N., & Pattatucci, A. M. L. (1993). A linkage between DNA markers on the X chromosome and male sexual orientation. *Science, 261*: 321–327.

Harding, C. (2001). Introduction: Making sense of sexuality. In: C. Harding (Ed.), *Sexuality: Psychoanalytic Perspectives* (pp. 1–17). Hove: Brunner-Routledge.

Harry, J. (1983). Parasuicide, gender, and gender deviance. *Journal of Health and Social Behavior, 24*: 350–361.

Haynal, A. (1968). Le syndrome de couvade (et contribution à la psychologie et psychopathologie de l'homme en face de la reproduction). *Annales Médico-Psychologiques, 126* (4): 539–571.

Haynal, A. (1974). Geschlechtsidentität und ihre Störungen. *Sexualmedizin, 3*: 111–114.

Haynal, A. (1977). Men facing reproduction. *Dynamische Psychiatrie, 10*: 360–368.

Heinemann, E. (1998). "Fakafefine": Männer, die wie Frauen sind: Inzesttabu und Transsexualität in Tonga (Polynesien). *Psyche, 52*: 473–498.

Herdt, G., & McClintock, M. (2000). The magical age of 10. *Archives of Sexual Behavior, 29* (6): 587–606.

Herold, R. (2004). Phantasie eines Geschlechtswechsels: Zur Psychoanalyse der Transsexualität. *Zeitschrift für Sexualforschung, 17*: 323–358.

Hertrampf, H. (1999). Phantastisch: Der gleiche Mensch, nur ein anderes Geschlecht. *Zeitschrift für Sexualforschung, 12*: 330–349.

Hines, M. (1998). Abnormal sexual development and psychosexual issues. *Baillieres Clinical Endocrinology and Metabolism, 12* (1): 173–189.

Hirschfeld, M. (1910). *Die Transvestiten: Eine Untersuchung über den erotischen Verkleidungstrieb mit umfangreichem casuistischem und historischem Material.* Berlin: Medizinischer Verlag.

Hirschfeld, M. (1923). Die intersexuelle Konstitution. *Jahrbuch für sexuelle Zwischenstufen, 23*: 3–27.

Hoffman, I. Z. (1998). *Ritual and spontaneity in the psychoanalytic process.* Hillsdale, NJ: Analytic Press.

Holt, R. R. (1992). The contemporary crisis of psychoanalysis. *Psychoanalysis and Contemporary Thought, 15*: 375–403.

Isay, R. A. (1989). *Being Homosexual: Gay Men and Their Development.* New York: Farrar, Straus, Giroux.

Isay, R. A. (1996). *Becoming Gay.* New York: Pantheon Books.

Jackson, P. L., & Decety, J. (2004). Motor cognition: A new paradigm to study self–other interactions. *Current Opinion in Neurobiology, 14*: 259–263.

*Janssen, P. L. (1984). Zum transsexuellen Symptom in einem Partnerarrangement—Nur ein Fall? *Zeitschrift für Psychotherapie und Medizinische Psychologie, 34*: 76–80.

Jimenez, J. P. (2004). A psychoanalytical phenomenology of perversion. *International Journal of Psychoanalysis, 85*: 65–82.

Joseph, B. (1985). Transference: The total situation. *International Journal of Psychoanalysis, 66*: 447–454.

Kagan, J. (1989). *Unstable ideas: Temperament, Cognition and Self.* Cambridge, MA: Harvard University Press.

Kallman, F. J. (1952a). *Heredity in Health and Mental Disorder: Principles of Psychiatric Genetics in the Light of Comparative Twin Studies.* New York: Norton.

Kallman, F. J. (1952b). Twin and sibship study of overt male homosexuality. *American Journal of Human Genetics, 4*: 136–146.

Kandel, E. R. (1999). Biology and the future of psychoanalysis: A new intellectual framework for psychiatry revisited. *American Journal of Psychiatry, 156*: 505–524.

Kaplan-Solms, K., & Solms, M. (2000). *Clinical Studies in Neuro-Psychoanalysis.* London: Karnac.

Kendler, K. S., Thornton, L. M., Gilman, S. E., & Kessler, R. C. (2000). Sexual orientation in a U.S. national sample of twin and nontwin sibling pairs. *American Journal of Psychiatry, 157*: 1843–1846.

*Kernberg, O. (1975). *Borderline-Störungen und pathologischer Narzißmus.* Frankfurt a.M.: Suhrkamp, 1978.

Kernberg, O. (1976). *Object Relations Theory and Clinical Psychoanalysis.* New York: Aronson.

Kernberg, O. (1985). Ein konzeptuelles Modell zur männlichen Perversion. *Forum der Psychoanalyse, 1*: 167–189.

Kernberg, O. (1991a). Aggression and love in the relationship of the couple. *Journal of the American Psychoanalytic Association, 39*: 45–70.

Kernberg, O. (1991b). Sadomasochism: Sexual excitement and perversion. *Journal of the American Psychoanalytic Association, 39*: 333–362.

Kernberg, O. (1991c). Sexual excitement and rage. *Sigmund Freud House Bulletin, 15*: 3–38.

Kernberg, O. (1992). *Aggression in Personality Disorders and Perversions.* New Haven, CT/London: Yale University Press.

Kernberg, O. (1995). *Love Relations: Normality and Pathology.* New Haven, CT/London: Yale University Press.

Kessler, S., & McKenna, W. (1985). *Gender: An Ethnomethodological Approach.* Chicago, IL: University of Chicago Press.

Khan, M. M. R. (1979). *Alienation in Perversions.* London: Karnac, 1989. [German: *Entfremdung bei Perversionen.* Frankfurt a.M.: Suhrkamp, 1984.]

*King, D. (1986). "The transvestite and the transsexual: A case study of public categories and private identities." PhD dissertation, University of Essex.

King, P., & Steiner, R. (Eds.) (1991). *The Freud-Klein Controversies 1941–45.* London/New York: Tavistock, Routledge.

Kinsey, A., Pomeroy, W., & Martin, C. (1948). *Sexual Behavior in the Human Male.* Philadelphia, PA: Saunders.

Kinsey, A., Pomeroy, W., & Martin, C. (1953). *Sexual Behavior in the Human Female.* Philadelphia, PA: Saunders.

Kirkpatrick, M., & Friedmann, C. (1976). Treatment of requests for sex-change surgery with psychotherapy. *American Journal of Psychiatry, 133*: 1194–1196.

Klein, M., Heimann, P., Isaacs, S., & Riviere, J. (Eds.) (1946). *Developments in Psychoanalysis.* London: Hogarth Press.

Klein, M. (1961). *Narrative of a Child Analysis.* London: Hogarth Press.

Köhler, L. (1998). Einführung in die Entstehung des Gedächtnisses. In: M. Koukkou, M. Leuzinger-Bohleber, & W. Mertens (Eds.), *Erinnerte Wirklichkeiten: Zum Dialog zwischen Psychoanalyse und Neurowissenschaften, Vol. 1* (pp. 131–223). Stuttgart: Verlag Internationale Psychoanalyse.

Kohon, G. (Ed.) (1999). *The Dead Mother. The Work of André Green.* London: Routledge.

Kohut, H. (1971). *Narzißmus.* Frankfurt a.M.: Suhrkamp, 1973.

*Krapf, E. E. (1956). Cold and warmth in the transference experience. *International Journal of Psychoanalysis, 37*: 381–394.

Krause, R. (1983). Zur Onto- und Phylogenese des Affektsystems und ihrer Beziehungen zu psychischen Störungen. *Psyche, 37*: 1015–1043.

Krause, R. (1991). Zur Psychodynamik der Emotionsstörungen. In: K. Scherer (Ed.), *Enzyklopädie der Psychologie, Vol. C/IV/*3: *Emotionen* (pp. 630–705). Göttingen: Hogrefe.

Krause, R. (1992). Die Zweierbeziehung als Grundlage der psychoanalytischen Therapie. *Psyche, 46*: 588–612.

Krause, R. (2000). Emotionsstörungen. In: J. H. Otto, H. A. Euler, & H. Mandl (Eds.), *Emotionspsychologie: Ein Handbuch.* Weinheim: Beltz.

Krause, R., Steimer-Krause, E., & Ullrich, B. (1992). Use of affect research in dynamic psycho-therapy. In: M. Leuzinger-Bohleber, H. Schneider, & R. Pfeifer (Eds.), *Two Butterflies on My Head: Psychoanalysis in the Scientific Dialogue* (pp. 277–292). Berlin/Heidelberg/New York: Springer.

Krause, R., Steimer-Krause, E., & Burkhard, U. (1992). Anwendung der Affektforschung auf die psychoanalytisch-psychotherapeutische Praxis. *Forum der Psychoanalyse, 8*: 238–253.

Kruijver, F. (2004). "Sex in the brain. Gender differences in the human hypothalamus and adjacent areas. Relationship to transsexualism, sexual orientation, sex hormone receptors and endocrine status." PhD dissertation, University of Amsterdam.

Kubie, L. S., & Mackie, J. B. (1968). Clinical issues raised by operation for gender transmutations. *Journal of Nervous and Mental Diseases, 147*: 431–444.

Kubie, L. S. (1974). The drive to become both sexes. *Psychoanalytic Quarterly, 43*: 349–426.

Küchenhoff, B. (1988). Transsexualismus als Symptom. *Nervenarzt, 59*: 734–738.

Lacan, J. (1954). *The Seminar of Jacques Lacan. Book I: Freud's Papers on Technique,* ed. J.-A. Miller, transl. J. Forrester. New York: Norton, 1988.

*Langer, D. (1985). Der Transsexuelle: Eine Herausforderung für die Kooperation zwischen psychologischer und chirurgischer Medizin. *Fortschritte der Neurologie Psychiatrie, 53*: 67–84.

Laplanche, J. (1988). *Die allgemeine Verführungstheorie und andere Aufsätze.* Tübingen: Edition diskord.

Laplanche, J. (1995). Seduction, persecution, revelation. *International Journal of Psychoanalysis, 76*: 663–682.

Laplanche, J. (2001). Sexuality and attachment in metapsychology. In: D. Widlöcher (Ed.), *Infantile Sexuality and Attachment* (pp. 37–54). New York: Other Press.

Laplanche, J., & Pontalis, J. B. (1968). Fantasy and the origins of sexuality. *International Journal of Psychoanalysis, 49*: 1–19.

Laub, D., Peskin, H., & Auerhahn, N. C. (1995). Der zweite Holocaust: Das Leben ist bedrohlich. *Psyche, 49*: 18–40.

Laumann, E. O., Gagnon, J. H., Michael, R. T., & Michaels, S. (1994). *The Social Organization of Sexuality: Sexual Practices in the United States.* Chicago, IL: University of Chicago Press.

Lazarus, R. S. (1993). From psychological stress to the emotions: A history of changing outlooks. *Annual Review of Psychology, 44*: 1–121.

Leuzinger-Bohleber, M. (1984). Transvestitische Symptombildung. Klinischer Beitrag zur Ätiologie, Psychodynamik und Analysierbarkeit transvestitischer Patienten. *Psyche, 18*: 817–847.

Leuzinger-Bohleber, M. (1987). *Veränderung kognitiver Prozesse in Psychoanalysen. Vol. 1: Eine hypothesengenerierende Einzelfallstudie.* Berlin/New York/Tokyo: Springer (PSZ).

Leuzinger-Bohleber, M. (1989). *Veränderung kognitiver Prozesse in Psychoana-*

lysen. Vol. 2: Fünf aggregierte Einzelfallstudien. Berlin/New York/Tokyo: Springer (PSZ).

Leuzinger-Bohleber, M. (2001). The "Medea fantasy": An unconscious determinant of psychogenic sterility. *International Journal of Psychoanalysis, 82*: 323–345.

Leuzinger-Bohleber, M. (2002). Die langen Schatten von Krieg und Verfolgung: Kriegskinder in Psychoanalysen. *Psyche, 57*: 982–1016.

Leuzinger-Bohleber, M., & Bürgin, D. (2003). Pluralism and unity in psychoanalytic research: Some introductory remarks. In: M. Leuzinger-Bohleber, A. U. Dreher, & J. Canestri (Eds.), *Pluralism and Unity? Methods of Research in Psychoanalysis* (pp. 1–25). London: International Psychoanalytical Association.

Leuzinger-Bohleber, M., Dreher, A. U., & Canestri, J. (Eds.) (2003). *Pluralism and Unity? Methods of Research in Psychoanalysis.* London: International Psychoanalytical Association.

Leuzinger-Bohleber, M., Fischmann, T., & Research Committee for Conceptual Research (in press). What is conceptual research in psychoanalysis. *International Journal of Psychoanalysis.*

Leuzinger-Bohleber, M., & Kächele, H. (1988). From Calvin to Freud: Using an artificial intelligence model to investigate cognitive changes during psychoanalysis. In: H. Dahl, H. Kächele, & H. Thomä (Eds.), *Psychoanalytic Process Research Strategies* (pp. 291–397). Berlin/New York/Tokyo: Springer.

Leuzinger-Bohleber, M., & Pfeifer, R. (1998). Erinnerung in der Übertragung—Vergangenheit in der Gegenwart? Psychoanalyse und Embodied Cognitive Science: Ein interdisziplinärer Dialog zum Gedächtnis. *Psyche-Z. Psychoanal., 52*: 884–919.

Leuzinger-Bohleber, M., & Pfeifer, R. (2002). Remembering a depressive primary object: Memory in the dialogue between psychoanalysis and Cognitive Science. *International Journal of Psychoanalysis, 83*: 3–33.

Leuzinger-Bohleber, M., Schneider, H., & Pfeifer, R. (Eds.) (1992). *"Two Butterflies on My Head . . ." Psychoanalysis in the Interdisciplinary Scientific Dialogue.* Berlin/New York/Tokyo: Springer.

Lewes, K. (1988). *The Psychoanalytic Theory of Male Homosexuality.* New York: Simon & Schuster.

Lewis, M., & Brooks-Gunn, J. (1979). *Social Cognition and the Acquisition of Self.* New York: Plenum Press.

Lewis, M. D. (1963). A case of transvestism with multiple body-phallus identification. *International Journal of Psychoanalysis, 44*: 345–351.

Lichtenstein, H. (1977). Identity and sexuality. In: *The Dilemma of Human Identity* (pp. 49–122). New York: Aronson.

Limentani, A. (1979). The significance of transsexualism in relation to some basic psychoanalytic concepts. *International Review of Psychoanalysis, 6*: 139–153.

Lincke, H. (1981). *Instinktverlust und Symbolbildung.* Berlin: Severin.

Linday, L. (1994). Maternal reports of pregnancy, genital, and related fantasies in preschool and kindergarten children. *Journal of the American Academy of Child and Adolescent Psychiatry, 33*: 416–423.

Loewald, H. W. (1960). On the therapeutic action of psycho-analysis. *International Journal of Psychoanalysis, 41*, 16–33.

Lothstein, L. (1977). Psychotherapy with patients with gender dysphoria syndromes. *Bulletin of the Menninger Clinic, 41*: 563–582.

Lothstein, L. (1983). *Female-to-Male Transsexualism.* Boston, MA/London: Routledge.

Lothstein, L., & Levine, S. B. (1981). Expressive psychotherapy with gender-dysphoric patients. *Archives of General Psychiatry, 38*: 924–929.

Luca, M. (2002). Containment of the sexualized and erotized transference. *Journal of Clinical Psychoanalysis, 11*: 648–662.

Maccoby, E. E. (1998). *The Two Sexes: Growing Up Apart, Coming Together.* Cambridge, MA: Harvard University Press.

Maccoby, E. E., & Jacklin, C. N. (1974). *The Psychology of Sex Differences.* Palo Alto, CA: Stanford University Press.

Mahler, M., Pine, F., & Bergman, A. (1975). *The Psychological Birth of the Human Infant.* New York: Basic Books.

Main, M., & Hesse, E. (1990). Parents' unresolved traumatic experience are related to infant disorganized attachment status: Is frightened and/or frightening parental behavior the linking mechanism? In: M. T. Greenberg, D. Cicchetti, & E. M. Commings (Eds.), *Attachment in Preschool Years: Theory, Research, and Intervention* (pp. 161–184). Chicago, IL: University of Chicago Press.

Malyon, A. K. (1982). Psychotherapeutic implications of internalized homophobia in gay men. *Journal of Homosexuality, 7*: 59–69.

Mann, D. (1997). *Psychotherapy: An Erotic Relationship. Transference and Countertransference Passions.* London: Routledge.

Marantz, S., & Coates, S. (1991). Mothers of boys with gender identity disorder: A comparison to normal controls. *Journal of the American Academy of Child and Adolescent Psychiatry, 30*: 136–143.

Masters, W., & Johnson, V. (1966). *Human Sexual Response.* Boston, MA: Little, Brown.

Masters, W., & Johnson, V. (1970). *Human Sexual Inadequacy.* Boston, MA: Little, Brown.

Matt, P. von (1989). *Liebesverrat. Die Treulosen in der Literatur.* Munich: Deutscher Taschenbuch Verlag, 1998.

Mayes, L. C. (2005). "Revisiting the concept of parental preoccupation: Genes, neural circuits and experiential contributions to parental behaviour." Paper presented at the Research Associates of the American Psychoanalytic Association, Annual Meeting of American Psychoanalytic Association, New York City (22 January).

*McCarroll, H. (1999). Performativity, transsexualism, and benevolent psychopathology. *Psychoanalytic Dialogues, 9*: 505–530.

McConaghy, N. (1993). *Sexual Behavior: Problems and Management.* New York/ London: Plenum Press.

McDougall, J. (1986). Identifications, neo-needs and neo-sexualities. *International Journal of Psychoanalysis, 67*: 19.

McDougall, J. (1995). *The Many Faces of Eros: A Psychoanalytic Exploration of Human Sexuality.* London: Free Association Books.

McEwen, B. S. (1983). Gonadal steroid influences on brain development and sexual differentiation. In: R. O. Greep (Ed.), *Reproductive Physiology, Vol. 4: International Review of Physiology* (pp. 99–145). Baltimore, MD: University Park Press.

*Mead, M. (1949). *Male and Female.* New York: Morrow.

Meaney, M. J. (1989). The sexual differentiation of social play. *Psychiatric Development, 3*: 247–261.

Meaney, M. J., Stewart, J., & Beatty, W. W. (1985). Sex differences in social play: The socialization of sex roles. In: J. S. Rosenblatt, C. Bear, C. M. Busnell, & P. Plater (Eds.), *Advances in the Study of Behavior, Vol. 15.* San Diego, CA: Academic Press.

Merten, J. (2001). *Beziehungsregulation in Psychotherapien. Maladaptive Beziehungsmuster und der therapeutische Prozeß.* Stuttgart: Kohlhammer.

Merten, J., & Krause, R. (2003). What makes good therapists fail? In: P. Philippot, E. J. Coats, & R. S. Feldman (Eds.), *Nonverbal Behaviour in Clinical Settings.* Oxford: Oxford University Press.

Mertens, W. (1998). Aspekte der psychoanalytischen Gedächtnistheorie. In: M. Koukkou, M. Leuzinger-Bohleber, & W. Mertens (Eds.), *Erinnerte Wirklichkeiten: Zum Dialog zwischen Psychoanalyse und Neurowissenschaften, Vol. 1* (pp. 48–130). Stuttgart: Verlag Internationale Psychoanalyse.

Meyenburg, B. (1992). Aus der Psychotherapie eines transsexuellen Patienten. *Zeitschrift für Sexualforschung, 5*: 95–110.

*Meyer, J. K. (1996). Sexualities and homosexualities. *Psychoanalytic Quarterly, 65*: 830–832.

Meyer-Bahlburg, H. F. L. (1994). Intersexuality and the diagnosis of gender identity disorder. *Archives of Sexual Behavior, 23*: 21–40.

Michaels, A. (1996). *Fugitive Pieces.* Toronto: McClelland & Stewart.

Mitchell, S. A. (1988). *Relational Concepts in Psychoanalysis: An Integration.* Cambridge, MA: Harvard University Press.

Mitchell, S. A. (2002). *Can Love Last? The Fate of Romance over Time.* New York: Norton.

Mitscherlich, A. (1950–51). 66. Wanderversammlung der Südwestdeutschen Psychiater und Neurologen, Badenweiler, 2–3. June 1950. Erstes Leitthema: Daseinsanalyse. *Psyche, 4*: 226–234.

Mitscherlich, A., Bally, G., Binder, H., Binswanger, L., Bleuler, M., Brun, R., Dührssen, A., Gollner, W. E., Jores, A., Jung, C. G., Kranz, H., Kemper, W., Meng, H., Mohr, F., Müller, M., Schultz-Hencke, H., Seitz, W., Staehelin, J. E., Steck, H., & Weizsäcker, V. v. (1950–51a). a. Rundfrage über ein Referat auf der 66. Wanderversammlung der Südwestdeutschen Psychiater und Neurologen in Badenweiler. *Psyche, 4*: 448–477.

Mitscherlich, A., Georgi, F., Göppert, H., Gundert, H., Mauz, F., Zutt, J., & Boss, M. (1950–51b). b. Rundfrage über ein Referat auf der 66. Wanderversammlung der Südwestdeutschen Psychiater und Neurologen in Badenweiler. *Psyche, 4*: 626–640.

Modell, A. H. (1984). *Psychoanalysis in a New Context.* New York: International Universities Press.

Money, J., Hampson, J. G., & Hampson, J. L. (1955a). Hermaphroditism: Recommodations concerning assignment of sex, change of sex, and psychologic management. *Bulletin of Johns Hopkins Hospital, 97*: 284–300.

Money, J., Hampson, J. G., & Hampson, J. L. (1955b). An examination of some basic sexual concepts: The evidence of human hermaphroditism. *Bulletin of Johns Hopkins Hospital, 97*: 301–310.

Money, J., Hampson, J. G., & Hampson, J. L. (1956). Sexual incongruitis and psychopathology: The evidence of human hermaphroditism. *Bulletin of Johns Hopkins Hospital, 98*: 43–57.

Morgenthaler, F. (1974). Zur Theorie und Therapie von Perversionen. *Psyche, 28*: 1077–1099.

Morgenthaler, F. (1984). *Homosexualität, Heterosexualität, Perversion.* Frankfurt: Qumram.

Moser, U., von Zeppelin, I., & Schneider, W. (1991). Computer-simulation of a model of neurotic defense processes. In: U. Moser & I. von Zeppelin (Eds.), *Cognitive and Affective Processes: New Ways of Psychoanalytic Modelling* (pp. 23–40). Berlin/Heidelberg/New York: Springer.

Moyer, K. E. (Ed.) (1976). *Physiology of Aggression.* New York: Raven Press.

Novick, J., & Novick, K. K. (1991). Some comments on masochism and the delusion of omnipotence from a developmental perspective. *Journal of the American Psychoanalytic Association, 39*: 307–332.

Ogden, T. H. (1989). *The Primitive Edge of Experience.* Hillsdale, NJ/London, Jason Aronson.

Oppenheimer, A. (1989). Le refus du masculine dans l'agir transsexual. *Adolescence, 7*: 155–169.

Oppenheimer, A. (1991). The wish for a sex-change: A challenge to psychoanalysis? *International Journal of Psychoanalysis, 72*: 221–232.

*Ovesey, L., & Person, E. (1973). Gender identity and sexual psychopathology in men: A psychodynamic analysis of homosexuality, transsexualism and transvestism. *Journal of the American Academy of Psychoanalysis,* 1: 53–72.

*Ovesey, L., & Person, E. (1976). Transvestism: A disorder of the sense of self. *International Journal of Psychoanalytic Psychotherapy, 5*: 219–235.

Panksepp, J. (1998). *Affective neuroscience.* New York: Oxford University Press.

Paul, J. P. (1993). Childhood cross-gender behavior and adult homosexuality: The resurgence of biological models of sexuality. *Journal of Homosexuality, 24*: 41–54.

Pelligrini, A. D., & Smith, P. I. (1998). Physical activity play: The nature and functions of a neglected aspect of play. *Child Development, 69*: 577–598.

Person, E. (1976). Discussion. Initiation fantasies and transvestism. *Journal of the American Psychoanalytic Association, 24*: 547–553.

Person, E. (1995). *By Force of Fantasy*. New York: Basics Books.

Person, E. (2001). Response to Juliet Mitchell's reflections. *Studies in Gender and Sexuality, 2*: 261–275.

*Person, E., & Ovesey, L. (1973). The psychodynamics of male transsexualism. In: R. Friedmann (Ed.), *Sex Differences in Behavior* (pp. 315–325). New York.

Person, E., & Ovesey, L. (1974a). The transsexual syndrome in males. I. Primary transsexualism. *American Journal of Psychotherapy, 28*: 4–20.

Person, E., & Ovesey, L. (1974b). The transsexual syndrome in males. II. Secondary transsexualism. *American Journal of Psychotherapy, 28*: 174–193.

*Person, E., & Ovesey, L. (1978). Transvestism: New perspectives. *Journal of the American Academy of Psychoanalysis, 6*: 301–324.

Person, E., & Ovesey, L. (1993). Psychoanalytische Theorien zur Geschlechtsidentität. *Psyche, 47*: 504–529.

Pfäfflin, F. (1983). Probleme der psychotherapeutischen Behandlung transsexueller Patienten. *Psychotherapie, Psychosomatik, Medizinische Psychologie, 3*: 89–92.

Pfäfflin, F. (1992). Regrets after sex reassignment surgery. *Journal of Psychology and Human Sexuality, 5*: 69–85.

Pfäfflin, F. (1993). *Transsexualität*. Stuttgart: Enke.

Pfäfflin, F. (1994). Zur transsexuellen Abwehr. *Psyche, 48*: 904–931.

Pfäfflin, F. (1997). Sex reassignment, Harry Benjamin, and some European roots. *International Journal of Transgenderism, 1* (2) (http: www.symposion.com/ijt/ijtco2o2.htm).

Pfäfflin, F. (2003). Understanding transgendered phenomena. In: S. Levine (Ed), *Handbook of Clinical Sexuality for Mental Health Professionals* (pp. 291–310). New York/Hove: Brunner-Routledge.

*Pfäfflin, F., & Junge, A. (Eds.) (1992a). *Geschlechtsumwandlung. Abhandlungen zur Transsexualität*. Stuttgart/New York: Schattauer.

Pfäfflin, F., & Junge, A. (1992b). Nachuntersuchungen nach Geschlechtsumwandlung. In: F. Pfäfflin & A. Junge (Eds), *Geschlechtsumwandlung. Abhandlungen zur Transsexualität* (pp. 149–457). Stuttgart/New York: Schattauer.

Pfäfflin, F., & Junge, A. (1998). Sex reassignment: Thirty years of international follow-up studies. A comprehensive review, 1961–1991. *International Journal of Transgenderism, book section* (http: www.symposion.com/ijt/books/index.htm).

Pfeifer, R., & Leuzinger-Bohleber, M. (1986). Application of cognitive science methods to psychoanalysis: A case study and some theory. *International Review of Psycho-Analysis, 13*: 221–240.

Pfeifer, R., & Scheier, C. (1999). *Understanding Intelligence*. Cambridge, MA: MIT Press.

Phillips, S. H. (2003). Homosexuality: Coming out of the confusion. *International Journal of Psychoanalysis, 84*: 1431–1450.

Phillips, S. H. (2004). Reply to Drs. Friedman and Downey. *International Journal of Psychoanalysis, 85*: 523–524.

Pizer, S. (1998). *Building Bridges: The Negotiation of Paradox in Psychoanalysis.* Hillsdale, NJ: Analytic Press.

Portman, L., Hale, R., & Campbell, D. (2005). "What we know and what we don't know about paedophilia." Paper presented at the Sixth Joseph Sandler Research Conference, Sexual Deviation: 100 Years after Freud's *Three Essays on the Theory of Sexuality*, London (March).

Prince, V. (1978). *Understanding Cross Dressing.* Los Angeles, CA: Chevalier.

Prus, R. (1997). *Subcultural Mosaics and Intersubjective Realities: An Ethnographic Research Agenda for Pragmatizing the Social Sciences.* Albany, NY: State University of New York Press.

Quinodoz, D. (1998). A fe/male transsexual patient in psychoanalysis. *International Journal of Psychoanalysis, 79*: 95–111.

Quinodoz, D. (1999). Ein/e transsexuelle/r Patient/in in Psychoanalyse. *Zeitschrift für Sexualforschung, 12*: 287–307.

Quinodoz, D. (2002). Temination of a fe/male transsexual patient's analysis. An example of general validity. *International Journal of Psychoanalysis, 83*: 783–798.

Ramachandran, V. S. (1998). *Phantoms in the Brain: Probing the Mysteries of the Human Brain.* New York: Morrow.

Rapaport, D. (1960). On the psychoanalytic theory of motivation. In: *Col- lected Papers of David Rapaport* (pp. 853–915). New York: Basic Books, 1967.

*Raymond, J. (1979). *The Transsexual Empire.* Boston, MA: Beacon Press.

Reiche, R. (1984). Sexualität, Identität, Transsexualität. *Beiträge zur Sexualforschung, 59*: 51–64. [Also in: M. Dannecker & V. Sigusch (Eds.), *Sexualtheorie und Sexualpolitik* (pp. 51–64). Stuttgart: Enke.]

Reik, T. (1914). Couvade. *Imago.* [Reprinted in: *Ritual, Psycho-analytic Studies.* New York, International Universities Press, 1958.]

Rice, G., Anderson, C., Risch, N., & Ebers, G. (1995). "Male homosexuality: Absence of linkage to micro satellite markers on the X-chromosome in a Canadian study." Paper presented at the Annual Meeting of the International Academy of Sex Research, Provincetown, MA.

*Richter-Appelt, H. (2003). Psychotherapie bei Störungen der Geschlechtsidentität. In: G. Poscheschnik, K. Ernst, & Klagenfurter Psychoanalytische Mittwoch-Gesellschaft (Eds.), *Psychoanalyse im Spannungsfeld von Humanwissenschaft, Therapie und Kulturtheorie* (pp. 165–175). Frankfurt a.M.: Brandes u. Apsel.

Riedl, R. (1981). *Biologie der Erkenntnis. Die stammesgeschichtlichen Grundlagen der Vernunft* (pp. 52–77). Berlin: Parey.

Roiphe, H., & Galenson, E. (1981). *Infantile Origins of Sexual Identity.* New York: International Universities Press.

Rosenfeld, D. (1984). Hypochondrias, somatic delusion and body schema in psychoanalytic practice. *International Journal of Psychoanalysis, 65*: 377–387.

Rosenfeld, H. (1952). Transference phenomena and transference analysis in an acute catatonic schizophrenic patient. *International Journal of Psychoanalysis, 33*, 457–464.

*Rosenfield, I. (1988). *The Intervention of Memory.* New York: Basic Books.

*Ross, J. M. (1975). The development of paternal identity: A critical review of the literature on nurturance and generativity in boys and men. *Journal of the American Psychoanalytic Association, 23*: 783–817.

Roth, G. (2001). *Fühlen, Denken, Handeln: Wie das Gehirn unser Verhalten steuert.* Frankfurt a.M.: Suhrkamp.

Roughton, R. (1995a). Overcoming antihomosexual bias: A progress report. *The American Psychoanalyst, 29* (4): 15–16.

Roughton, R. (1995b). Action and acting out. In: B. E. Moore & B. D. Fine (Eds.), *Psychoanalysis: The Basic Concepts* (pp. 130–145). New Haven, CT: Yale University Press.

*Runte, A. (1999). Zeichen des Geschlechts: Die Rolle des Diskurses bei der (Re-)Konstruktion von Transsexualität. *Zeitschrift der Semiotik, 21*: 325–348.

Sandberg, D. E., Meyer-Bahlburg, H. F. L., Ehrhardt, A. A., & Yager, T. J. (1993). The prevalence of gender-atypical behavior in elementary school children. *Journal of the American Academy of Child and Adolescent Psychiatry, 32*: 306–314.

Sandell, R., Blomberg, J., Lazar, A., Carlsson, J., Broberg, J. & Schubert, J. (2000). Varieties of long-term outcome among patients in psychoanalysis and long-term psychotherapy. *International Journal of Psychoanalysis, 81*: 921–942

Sanders, A. R. (1998). Poster Presentation, 149th Annual Meeting of American Psychiatric Association, Toronto, Ontario, Canada.

Sanders, J. (1934). Homosexueele tweelingen nederl genesk. *Nederl. Tijdschrift voor Geneeskunde, 78*: 3346–3352.

*Sandler, J. (1960). The background of safety. *International Journal of Psychoanalysis, 41*: 352–356.

Sandler, J. (1976). Countertransference and role-responsiveness. *International Review of Psycho-Analysis, 3*: 43–47.

Sandler, J., & Dreher, A. U. (1991). An approach to conceptual research in psychoanalysis illustrated by a consideration of psychic trauma. *International Review of Psycho-Analysis, 18*: 133–141.

Sandler, J., Green, A., & Stern, D. N. (Eds.) (2000). *Clinical and Observational Psychoanalytic Research: Roots of a Controversy.* London: Karnac.

Sass, H., Wittchen, H. U., & Zaudig, M. (1996). *Diagnostisches und statistisches Manual psychischer Störungen, DSM-IV.* Göttingen: Hogrefe.

Schäppi, R. (1998). Les origines de l'intrication du sexuel et du social: Esquisse d'une phylogenèse. In: M.-T. Neyraut-Sutterman (Ed.), *L'animal et le psychanalyste: Le meurtre du grand singe.* Paris: L'Harmattan.

Schepanck, H. (1987). *Psychogene Erkrankungen der Stadtbevölkerung (epidemiologische und tiefenpsychologische Feldstudie)*. Heidelberg: Springer.

Schorsch, E. (1974). Phänomenologie der Transsexualität. Therapie: Geschlechtsumwandlung ohne Alternative. *Sexualmedizin, 3*: 195–198.

Schorsch, S., Galedary, G., Haag, A., Hauch, M., & Lohse, H. (1990). *Sex Offenders: Dynamics and Psychotherapeutic Strategies*. Berlin/New York/London: Springer.

Schwöbel, G. (1960a). Ein transvestitischer Mensch, die Bedeutung seiner Störungen und sein Wandel in der Psychoanalyse. *Schweizer Archiv für Neurologie und Psychiatrie, 86*: 358–382.

*Schwöbel, G. (1960b). *Psychosomatische Medizin*. Zürich: Rascher.

Searles, H. (1959). Oedipal love in the countertransference. *International Journal of Psychoanalysis, 40*: 180–190.

*Segal, M. M. (1965). Transvestism as an impulse and as a defence. *International Journal of Psychoanalysis, 46*: 209–217.

*Sidhar, A. P. (1978). Transvestism. *Samiksa, 32*: 87–94.

Sigusch, V. (1997). Transsexualismus: Forschungsstand und klinische Praxis. *Nervenarzt, 68*: 870–877.

Sigusch, V. (1998). Die neosexuelle Revolution: Über gesellschaftliche Transformationen der Sexualität in den letzten Jahrzehnten. *Psyche, 52*: 1192–1234.

Sigusch, V., Meyenburg, B., & Reiche, R. (1978). Transsexualität. *Sexualmedizin, 7*: 15–22, 107–116, 191–192.

Sigusch, V., Meyenburg, B., & Reiche, R. (1979). Transsexualität. In: V. Sigusch (Ed.), *Sexualität und Medizin* (pp. 249–311). Cologne: Kiepenheuer u. Witsch.

*Socarides, C. W. (1968). *Der offen Homosexuelle*. Frankfurt a.M.: Suhrkamp, 1971.

Socarides, C. W. (1970a). Pornography and perversions. *Archives of General Psychiatry, 22*: 490–498.

Socarides, C. W. (1970b). A psychoanalytic study of the desire for sexual transformation ("transsexualism"): The Plaster-of-Paris man. *International Journal of Psychoanalysis, 51*: 341–349.

Socarides, C. W. (1978). *Homosexuality*. New York: Jason Aronson.

Spence, D. P. (1982). *Narrative Truth and Historical Truth: Meaning and Interpretation in Psychoanalysis*. New York: Norton.

*Sperling, M. (1964). The analysis of a boy with transvestite tendencies. *Psychoanalytic Study of the Child, 19*: 204–231.

Spitz, R. (1945). Hospitalism: An inquiry into the genesis of psychiatric conditions in early childhood. *Psychoanalytic Study of the Child, 1*: 53–73.

Springer, A. (1981). *Pathologie der geschlechtlichen Identität. Transsexualismus und Homosexualität: Theorie, Klinik, Therapie*. Berlin/Heidelberg/Vienna/New York: Springer.

Spruiell, V. (1997). Review of the psychoanalytic theory of sexuality: Comments on the assault against it. *International Journal of Psychoanalysis, 78*: 357–361.

*Steffens, W., & Kächele, H. (1988). Abwehr und Bewältigung-Mechanismen und Strategien: Wie ist eine Integration möglich? In: H. Kächele & W. Steffens (Eds.), *Bewältigung und Abwehr. Beiträge zur Psychologie und Psychotherapie schwerer körperlicher Krankheiten* (pp. 1–50). Berlin/Heidelberg/New York: Springer.

Stein, R. (1995). Analysis of a case of transsexualism. *Psychoanalytic Dialogues, 5*: 257–289.

Stein, R. (1998a). The enigmatic dimension of sexual eperience: The "otherness" of sexuality and primal seduction. *Psychoanalytic Quarterly, 67*: 594–625.

Stein, R. (1998b). The poignant, the excessive and the enigmatic in sexuality. *International Journal of Psychoanalysis, 79*: 253–268.

Stein, R. (2005). Why perversion? False love and the perverse pact. *International Journal of Psychoanalysis, 86*: 775–801.

Steiner, J. (1993). *Psychic Retreats: Pathological Organisations in Psychotic, Neurotic, and Borderline Patients.* London/New York: Routledge.

Stern, D. (1985). *The Interpersonal World of the Infant: A View from Psychoanalysis and Developmental Psychology.* New York: Basic Books.

Stern, D. (1995). *The Motherhood Constellation.* New York: Basic Books.

Stoller, R. J. (1968). *Sex and Gender, Vol. 1: The Development of Masculinity and Femininity.* New York: Science House.

Stoller, R. J. (1969). Parental influences in male transsexualism. In: R. Green & J. Money (Eds.), *Transsexualism and Sex Reassignment* (pp. 153–169). Baltimore, MD: Johns Hopkins Press.

Stoller, R. J. (1973). *Splitting: A Case of Female Masculinity.* New York: Quadrangle.

Stoller, R. J. (1974). Foreword. In: R. Green, *Sexual Identity Conflict in Children and Adults* (pp. 9–14). New York: Basic Books.

Stoller, R. J. (1975a). *Perversion: The Erotic Form of Hatred.* London: Karnac, 1994. [German: *Perversion. Die erotische Form von Haß.* Reinbek: Rowohlt, 1979.]

Stoller, R. J. (1975b). Pornography and perversion. In: *Perversion: The Erotic Form of Hatred* (pp. 63–92). London: Karnac.

Stoller, R. J. (1975c). *The Transsexual Experiment: Sex and Gender, Vol. II.* London: Hogarth Press.

Stoller, R. J. (1979a). *Perversion, die erotische Form von Haß.* Reinbeck: Rowohlt.

Stoller, R. J. (1979b). *Sexual Excitement: Dynamics of Erotic Life.* New York: Pantheon.

Stoller, R. J. (1985a). *Observing the Erotic Imagination.* New Haven, CT: Yale University Press.

Stoller, R. J. (1985b). *Presentations of Gender.* New Haven, CT/London: Yale University Press.

*Stolorow, R. D. (1975). Appendum to a partial analysis of a perversion involving bugs: An illustration of the narcissistic function of perverse activity. *International Journal of Psychoanalysis, 56*: 361–364.

Strauss, A. (1993). *Continual Permutations of Action.* New York: Aldine de Gruyter.

Strauss, A. (Ed.) (1964). *The Social Psychology of G. H. Mead.* Chicago, IL: University of Chicago Press.

Sulloway, F. J. (1979). *Freud, Biologist of the Mind.* London: Burnett Books.

Suomi, S. J. (1991). Early stress and adult emotional reactivity in rhesus monkeys. In: *The Childhood Environment and Adult Disease* (pp. 171–188). (Ciba Foundation Symposium, No. 156, New Series.) New York: Wiley.

*Taylor, G. J. (1980). Splitting of the ego in transvestism and mask wearing. *International Review of Psychoanalysis, 7*: 511–520.

Terr, L. C. (1991). Between traumas: An outline and overview. *American Journal of Psychiatry, 148*: 10–20.

Thomä, H. (1957). Männlicher Transvestitismus und das Verlangen nach Geschlechtsumwandlung. *Psyche, 11*: 81–124.

Thomä, H., & Kächele, H. (1985). *Lehrbuch der psychoanalytischen Therapie.* Berlin: Springer.

Thorne, B. (1993). *Gender Play: Girls and Boys in School.* New Brunswick, NJ: Rutgers University Press.

Tinbergen, N. (1966). *Instinktlehre.* Berlin: Parey.

Tustin, F. (1981). *Autistic States in Children.* London: Routledge & Kegan Paul.

Varvin, S. (2003). Psychotherapy with a victim of extreme violence: Clinical case study and qualitative analysis. In: M. Leuzinger-Bohleber, A. H. Dreher, & J. Canestri (Eds.), *Pluralism and Unity: Methods of Research in Psychoanalysis* (168–183). London: The International Psychoanalytical Association.

Volkan, V. D. (1973). Transitional fantasies in the analysis of a narcissistic personality. *Journal of the American Psychoanalytic Association, 21*: 351–376.

*Volkan, V. D., & Masri, A. (1989). The development of female transsexualism. *American Journal of Psychotherapy, 43*: 92–107.

Walinder, J. (1967). *Transsexualism: A Study of Forty-Three Cases.* Göteborg: Akademieförlaget.

Wallerstein, R. S. (1988). One psychoanalysis or many? *International Journal of Psychoanalysis, 69*: 5–21.

Weinberg, G. (1972). *Society and the Healthy Homosexual.* New York: St. Martins Press.

*Weitzmann, E. L., Shamoian, C. A., & Golosow, N. (1970). Identity diffusion and the transsexual resolution. *Journal of Nervous and Mental Disease, 51*: 295–302.

Westen, D. (1997). Toward a clinically relevant and empirically sound theory of motivation. *International Journal of Psychoanalysis, 78*: 521–548.

Whitam, F. L., Diamond, M., & Martin, J. (1993). Homosexual orientation in twins: A report on 61 pairs and three triplet sets. *Archives of Sexual Behavior, 22*: 187–206.

Wiedeman, C. H. (1962). Survey of psychoanalytic literature on overt male homosexuality. *Journal of the American Psychoanalytic Association, 10*: 386–409.

Wiedeman, C. H. (1974). Homosexuality: A survey. *Journal of the American Psychoanalytic Association, 22*: 651–696.

Willick, M. S. (2001). Psychoanalysis and schizophrenia: A cautionary tale. *Journal of the American Psychoanalytic Association, 49*: 27–56.

Winnicott, D. W. (1956). Primary maternal preoccupation. In: *Collected Papers: Through Paediatrics to Psycho-Analysis.* London: Tavistock Publications.

Winnicott, D. W. (1960). *Maturational Processes and the Facilitating Environment.* New York: International Universities Press.

*Winnicott, D. W. (1971). *Playing and Reality.* London: Tavistock.

Winnicott, D. W. (1972). *Holding and Interpretation: Fragment of an Analysis.* London: Hogarth Press.

Winnicott, D. W. (1954). Metapsychological and clinical aspects of regression within the psycho-analytic set-up. In: D. W. Winnicott, *Through Paediatrics to Psycho-Analysis.* London: Hogarth Press, 1975.

Wolfe, S. (1990). "Psychopathology and psychodynamics of parents of boys with a gender identity disorder." PhD dissertation, City University of New York.

Young, R. M. (2001). Locating and relocating psychoanalytic ideas of sexuality. In: C. Harding (Ed.), *Sexuality: Psychoanalytic Perspectives* (pp. 18–34). Hove: Brunner-Routledge.

*Zavitzianos, G. (1977). The object in fetishism, homeovestism and transvestism. *International Journal of Psychoanalysis, 58*: 487–496.

Zhou, J., Hofman, M., Gooren, L., & Swaab, D. (1995). A sex difference in the human brain and its relation to transsexuality. *Nature, 378*: 68–70.

Zucker, K. J. (2004). Gender identity development and issues. *Child and Adolescent Psychiatric Clinics of North America, 13*: 551–568.

Zucker, K., & Bradley, S. (1995). *Gender Identity Disorder and Psychosexual Problems in Children and Adolescents.* New York: Guilford Press.

Zucker, K. J., Bradley, S. J., & Lowry Sullivan, C. B. (1996). Traits of separation anxiety in boys with gender identity disorder. *Journal of the American Academy of Child and Adolescent Psychiatry, 35*: 791–798.

Zucker, K. J., Bradley, S. J., & Sanikhani, M. (1997). Sex differences in referral rates of children with gender identity disorder: Some hypotheses. *Journal of Abnormal Child Psychology, 25*: 217–227.

INDEX

Made in the USA
Las Vegas, NV
19 September 2026

98121071-33bf-4599-801b-6671fa1d89b4R01